H3

D0866975

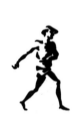

BY SUZY KALTER

Instant Parent
*The Complete Book of M*A*S*H*
How to Take Twenty Pounds Off Your Man

how to take 20 pounds off your man

by
SUZY KALTER

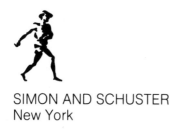

SIMON AND SCHUSTER
New York

Published by Simon and Schuster
A Division of Simon & Schuster, Inc.
Simon & Schuster Building
Rockefeller Center
1230 Avenue of the Americas
New York, New York 10020
SIMON AND SCHUSTER and colophon are registered
trademarks of Simon & Schuster, Inc.
Designed by Irving Perkins Associates
Manufactured in the United States of America

10 9 8 7 6 5 4 3 2 1

Library of Congress Cataloging in Publication Data

Kalter, Suzy.
  How to take 20 pounds off your man.

  1. Reducing. 2. Men—Healthandhygiene. I. Title.
II. Title: How to take twenty pounds off your man.
RM222.2.K24 1984   613.2′5   84-20248
ISBN 0-671-50618-8

Acknowledgments

I would like to thank my wonderful husband, Michael Gershman, without whom this book certainly would not have been possible!

Thanks also to Patricia Soliman, my editor; Pam Krauss, her assistant; and Joan Stewart, my friend and agent, who is planning to take twenty pounds off her husband any day now. Look out, Fred!

The text was checked for accuracy by Dr. Edward L. Singer; the introduction was written by my husband's physician, Dr. Howard Wilner—thank you both. Love and thanks also to Anne Gilbar and Dan Green.

To Aaron

CONTENTS

how
to
take 20 pounds
off your man

Foreword

I was pleased, flattered, and very surprised when Ms. Kalter asked me to write this foreword to her book. When I discovered that the subject of this tome was how to take weight off your husband, I was quite perplexed as well. For several years I have served as physician to Michael Gershman, the spouse of Ms. Kalter, and have been an abject failure in convincing him to lose weight. Despite all my efforts, the thin person screaming to be let out of his overweight body never made an appearance. Nevertheless, I consented to plow ahead and produce this foreword to a work designed to reduce the weight of American husbands.

Today, gourmet cooking and its natural by-product, eating, make up America's second fastest-growing pastime. Number one on the hit parade appears to be dieting. This has not always been so. I can remember when "children are starving in Africa," a phrase even more popular than "Where's the beef?" was used to encourage America's youth to consume all that was heaped on their plates. This Herculean effort produced over 200 million eaters in the United States and their number continued to grow into the 1950s. Following this proliferation, weight control and the diet industry began their ascendancy until now there are probably more dieters than eaters in these United States.

It has been estimated that several thousand diets have been published, and probably twice that number have been tried by the American public. Everything from the Beverly Hills Diet to the Drinking Man's Diet has tempted legions to reduce. Though the initial success rate is high, the long-term loss maintenance has proven dismal. Despite the use of modern techniques such as biofeedback, hypnotism, behavior modification, acupuncture, hospital-based eating-disorder centers, and so on, dieters continue to falter and fall by the wayside. In spite of the use of blue (non-fat) milk, sawdustlike bread, macrobiotic diets, and health food stores, this has been a disappointing era for the overweight.

I was therefore quite surprised and pleased to read this innovative book and discover how my patient and his wife succeeded. Ms. Kalter feels that most overweight Americans, including her husband, suffer from a problem with appetite, not hunger. She was able to take this suffering gentleman, "who quickly makes food 'all gone' more efficiently than a garbage disposal," and make him see the light. By the use of stealth, subterfuge, trick and treat, dieting with a partner, slogans such as "less is more," and visual aids such as "naked truth in the mirror test," Ms. Kalter was able to reduce Michael's weight by thirty-seven pounds. I suspect this success is in great part due to Michael's willing cooperation.

In my boyhood home, I was able to determine the day of the week by the main course at the dinner meal. Michael Gershman's diet was made more varied by the use of "veggies," including such delicacies as cactus leaves and fiddlehead ferns. He celebrates special occasions with crisp bacon and too-fatty duck, and gets goose only on Christmas. I have known for a long time that men are the privileged sex, but Ms. Kalter points out that once achieved, weight loss is more readily maintained by them.

I commend Ms. Kalter for her valiant efforts and success in the case of her husband and for this helpful, hopeful book. If you are a woman who loves a man, you will want to read this book and learn how to help your man to a new level of well-being.

HOWARD I. WILNER, M.D.

chapter **1**

A WOMAN'S WORK IS NEVER DONE

Why It Takes a Woman to Do a Man's Job

> Once made equal to man, a woman becomes
> his superior.
> —Socrates

Socrates said it all. I rest my case. Never under-
estimate the power of a woman, and all that.

Women just seem to be the stronger sex. As
such, they end up doing their own jobs—in the
offices or in the homes—and then subtly, carefully, delicately helping their husbands with yet
more tasks. Behind every great man, there's a
woman.

Sure, my husband lived for thirty-five years before he met me and possibly could have gone
another thirty-five without my help. But frankly,
I was worried about him. I thought he was a
walking case for General Hospital, a living dare
for Heart Attack City. I figured he'd kick the
bucket if he didn't lose some weight—and keep
it off. You've got the same worry about your man,
right? Probably with good reason.

17

Sure, his weight *should* be his responsibility. But in all the years you've known him, has he done anything either serious or lasting about it? Maybe he's been on diets before, but he's doubtless among the 85 percent of dieters who have lost and regained weight within the same year.

Although his health and his actual life span are being threatened by his weight, your Mr. Right has done little to help himself or to keep you from premature widowhood. You're concerned; he's oblivious?

It's time to take charge, woman.

Subtly, carefully, and delicately—of course. As is our wont.

The Problem According to Me

My life at home seems to be dedicated solely to two tasks:

- Getting my son to eat *something*
- Preventing my husband from eating *everything*

I don't worry too much about my son. Despite the fact that he eats one nourishing meal a week and seems to subsist merely on warm milk and white bread, chances are excellent that he will grow to be a wonderful person who will someday eat a full meal. I doubt he will ever be fat, since most slim children grow up to be slim adults.

My husband is a different story. He grew up in the chunky-size department and was still calling himself "pudgy" when we met—and he was thirty-five years old! Pudgy he was, indeed.

He had been thin once in his life. I know this because he gave me his army picture, and there he is, in black and white and stars and stripes, as thin as Uncle Sam. It might also be noted that most of his service to his country was performed from a hospital bed—he developed a bleeding ulcer—so the weight loss cannot be attributed to healthy eating or to being part of the lean, mean machine. He was never that thin again, although he did take off a good bit of weight when liquid protein diets were the rage. We had just moved to California, and he was loath to step into the apartment complex hot tub with his love handles hanging out. He went to a doctor, and carefully and steadily lost some thirty pounds. He drank only a white drink that looked something like a milk shake, ate steamed broccoli, and soon wore a size 36 trouser. I took a picture of him—fortunately with an instant camera, so I could get the image before he gained the weight back.

From our years together, and his forays into either diet or exercise, I knew he would never again be Army Thin. In fact, I finally realized he would never lose a pound unless I did something about it. Maybe it's the fact that I am an Aries, maybe it's because I'm just a pushy, aggressive, opinionated broad—but one day I merely decided that if *he* wasn't going to do something about his weight, by God, *I* would do something for him.

Men seem to put their energy into their careers first, and give whatever is left over to their families. Because the social pressures toward thinness are not nearly as great for men as they are for women, the average, slightly overweight American male rates his weight problem as a very low priority. Unless he is obese, his weight does not hinder his rise in the work force. Unless he is unduly fat and sloppy, he is able to woo you. The

health problems of being overweight are probably something he has so far been able to avoid by
ignoring them. While he knows he *should* shape
up, he'll think about it tomorrow just like that
famous philosopher, Scarlett O'Hara. To him, his
weight problem is *not* a problem.

A woman can gain three to five pounds and feel
"fat"; a man can gain forty to fifty pounds and
still be accepted by society as well groomed.
Good tailoring hides a multitude of sins. After all,
Luciano Pavarotti is considered a sex symbol. To
this day, when people tsk-tsk about John Belushi,
they mean drugs, not obesity. Few would consider calling John Houseman by his childhood
nickname, "Fat Jack." Men who are "fat" are
often termed "bearlike" or merely "big"—polite,
macho terms. When was the last time someone
politely called a woman "bearlike"? When was
the last time a woman gained forty or fifty pounds
and still thought she was sexy?

Women are used to dieting; despite the fact
that men can lose weight more easily than
women can, men are not. Women are used to the
pressures of Western culture that dictate, "Thin
is in." They needlepoint pillows announcing
their credo, "You can never be too rich or too
thin." (Men prefer slogans such as, "Yea, though
I walk through the Valley of the Shadow of
Death, I fear no evil . . . for I am the biggest son
of a bitch in the Valley.")

Even in our fitness-obsessed times, men, especially straight men, do not experience the pressure to be thin as poignantly as women do.
Married men over the age of thirty-five feel even
less pressure. Men diet every now and then
(often on a bet, which is a macho way of forcing

one to lose weight), suffer from the same yo-yo syndrome that affects women, and eventually rationalize their excess poundage with their masculinity. Until the day he dies, my husband will characterize his physical build as "big." Men think big is good.

As they age, men become more worried about their weight. Unfortunately they achieve this raised consciousness when they are forty-five to fifty, not twenty-five to thirty five, when it could make a serious difference. The new discovery that weight affects health only hits them when a friend of roughly the same age dies of a heart attack, or they themselves have a brush with mortality.

Most men like to think they are better equipped to deal with life's realities than their wives. I find that while they're busy running the ship, we're busy making sure it sails. My husband may think I'm disorganized, chatty, unmechanical, and scatterbrained (traits he is certain no man has ever possessed), but I happen to find him too unimaginative to realize the implications of his overweight state.

Okay, so I'm a bit of a female chauvinist. But listen to this: When Rita Rapp, the NASA dietician, was asked if she liked the astronauts "pantry" suggestion—that they take into space a loaded pantry so they could eat what they want when they want it—she replied, "My feeling is that it doesn't lead to good nutrition, in that they won't eat the right things." (This statement was made before there were women astronauts!) If the men who have the right stuff, whom we have chosen as national heroes and leaders of American society, cannot be trusted to eat the right foods, how can we expect our own husbands to do any better?

What's a wife to do? She can do what I did, what Rita Rapp does—take charge.

The women's movement has allowed us to leave the home and seek refuge in the working world. But we still return at night to most of the housework and mother-work. Gently forcing your man to lose weight can be just another of the little things you do for him—no different from sewing on his buttons, shortening his cuffs, or buying his shaving cream.

Man-Fat As a Feminist Issue

Why should you care about your husband's weight problem? Haven't you got enough on your hands, worrying about your own weight, and perhaps your children's? Isn't this just one more thing for you to be anxious about when you are overloaded as it is and have finally acknowledged that you don't have to be Superwoman? Well, life is hard. And harder still without a husband. New Year's Eve isn't that far away, and you don't want to have to start worrying about getting a date, do you?

I go by the old-fashioned notion that you married for better or for worse, and you certainly don't want to be left bereft, wrinkled, middle-aged, lonely, and possibly broke. Even if your house is paid for and the kids are safely through college, these are supposed to be the best years of your life, remember? These are the golden years you struggle to attain. If you plan on enjoying them together, you need a husband who is alive and well.

22

Taking twenty pounds off your husband—and keeping them off—will add years to his life, probably after age sixty-five. Perhaps those seem light-years away to you right now. But I assure you, if the good fairy came down on wings of sparkly gold on your husband's sixty-fifth birthday and asked you if you'd like your husband to live another five or ten years—you would jump at the chance.

Be selfish about it—it is in your own best interest for your husband to live as long as he possibly can. You don't want to have to take the garbage cans out yourself when you're sixty-two, do you?

The time to extend his life is now, not on his sixty-fifth birthday. Use the sensitivity, concern, and nurturing that women are famous for, and reap the benefits of having your man for as long as you can. Men traditionally die seven years earlier than women; if you are younger than your husband you may be facing a second marriage or a span of years when it would be nice to have a man around the house.

The Way to a Man's Heart Attack Is Through His Stomach

Mother was quick to point out, in all her postwar wisdom, that the way to a man's heart was through his stomach. She was wrong. That's the surest way to widowhood.

It took me eight years to figure out that I was killing my husband. Without ever serving *sauce béarnaise* or slathering mayonnaise on his onion dill whole wheat rolls, I was poisoning him by clogging his arteries and overworking his heart. A steak, a baked potato with butter and sour cream, some green beans with butter and toasted sesame seeds, a brown-and-serve roll or two, and a delicious treat from Sara Lee—the very foods my mother raised her family on, the same foods I had been taught to believe would make my marriage strong—were all it took.

One hundred million Americans have a weight problem. In men aged thirty to forty-nine, every extra pound means a 1 percent increase risk of dying within twenty-six years. In men aged fifty to sixty-two, each pound increases risk by 2 percent.

The leading cause of death among men is heart disease.

Cancer of the colon is the number-two killer and the most common form of cancer in America. Diet may be related.

If my husband died from any of these diseases because I was not careful in my food choices, I'd feel as guilty as Colonel Mustard in the billiard room with the rope. You just may be killing your husband without even knowing it.

Hereditary Troubles

Body type and a predisposition to certain diseases are inherited. You cannot change your husband's genetic code. But an incidence of heart disease in his family and a tendency toward overweight (especially in the shorter, pear-shaped, endomorph body type) should be a clear warning. You can ruin anyone's life by feeding him "bad" foods, but you are asking for a visit from the undertaker if you allow a man with a poor family history to gain weight.

A family history of early death and/or heart disease should be caution enough to keep your husband from eating dessert. Unfortunately, few people like to read the handwriting on the wall. My husband was so confident of his own immortality that he considered my prophecies of death and doom "hysterical outbreaks" and "overdramatic hogwash." Both of his parents dead before age sixty-five, and he tells me I'm overreacting!

A medical history is an important tool in prolonging life. (Many states now allow children placed for adoption to have full medical histories of their biological parents.) If you do not know your husband's family's history, make it your business to discover it, especially if he is ominously lacking in living relations. Heart disease and cancer, as well as many other diseases, run in families. Knowing of their existence can help you to save a life. The life you save will be your man's.

MEDICAL HISTORY

Name _____

Birthdate _____

Current Weight _____

Current medications taken on a regular basis _____

_____

Previous heart problems? (List date and treatment.) ___

_____

_____

Parents

Mother: Living?___Age (if dead, cite age at death)_____
Past illnesses, allergies, heart ailments, etcetera. Give
date and treatment if possible: _____

_____

_____

_____

Father: Living?___Age (if dead, cite age at death)_____
Past illnesses, allergies, heart ailments, etcetera. Give
date and treatment if possible: _____

_____

_____

_____

_____

If the information is available, include medical history of
grandparents, aunts and uncles, brothers and sisters.

Fat Passages

As mentioned, my husband was "pudgy" when
we met. I found his weight rather appealing. And
just as some women like to marry alcoholics and
then "cure" them, I was certain that under my
tender tutelage, Mike's weight would either remain stable or be reduced. I was wrong. He
gained steadily. And as he gained, I went through
a variety of psychological passages that Gail
Sheehy never encountered.

Stage One: Pleading, Begging, Sweet Talk

Mostly from parental pressure (my father is a doctor), I began sweetly to point out my husband's
two biggest medical problems:

- He smoked.
- He was overweight.

I begged him to tackle one or the other problem. I pleaded with him. I cajoled. I murmured sweet cautions in his ear. I gave up when I created so much tension that my marriage began to rock. I did not stop my father from having a few man-to-man talks with him. My husband reported back that I should get my father off his case. End of Stage One.

Stage Two: Enlisting Outside Help

If he didn't want to listen to me or my father, okay, that was his prerogative. I called his doctor. I applauded when his chiropractor said his back pain would ease if he lost thirty pounds. I went to exercise class with him, but the instructor made fun of him, so we quit.

Stage Three: Talking Tough

I was angry and afraid and downright disgusted and I told him so. Not only had pudgy given way to fat, but he refused to admit he had a problem or listen to anyone who could help. He ate like a pig. I mentioned it whenever possible. More tension. Adieu to our sex life.

Stage Four: Guilt

I kept thinking it was my fault. We should have found another exercise class. I should have bought Weight Watchers meals. I should have cooked the diet recipe my Mom sent me, the one where you substitute spaghetti squash for linguine. I must have done something wrong not to be able to break through to him. I was a bad wife.

Stage Five: Zen

I decided he had to do it for himself. You could drag a horse to water but you couldn't make him drink. It was his problem—not mine. I began to wonder who I would marry next time around.

Stage Six: Fury and Determination

Zen was bullshit. If he couldn't do it, *I* could do it for him.

I mention my stages because I later discovered that Dr. Kelly Bronwell at the University of Pennsylvania did a study on wives of overeaters and developed an eleven-phase cycle of feelings that is uncannily close to mine:

1. Minimization of the problem
2. Support for his new diets
3. Change in his food intake
4. Demand dieting
5. Harsh view of his body
6. Reproach
7. Comments to others
8. Self-blame
9. Resignation
10. Sarcasm and anger
11. Little hope of improvement

Maybe some women give up when they get to the end of Dr. Bronwell's list. After my short period of feeling sorry for myself, I had the most energy. I knew I could make my plan work. And I did. My husband now weighs 206 pounds, and the transition was nearly painless.

Two Can Tango (Maybe)

The plan in this book should be carried out by the whole family as a way of life. "Diets" that require one member of the family to eat a different kind of food, or to eat separately from the rest, never succeed. If your children need extra calories—a teenage boy who plays football after school may need 3,000 to 5,000 calories a day—or if you have no weight problem and care to indulge yourself, you can do the extra feeding or eating when your husband isn't watching. (After-school snacks were created to shovel in extra calories.) The basic plan is a family plan; it is a change to a healthier life-style and more healthful habits that, with luck, will be adapted and passed on from generation to generation—instead of heart trouble!

Because a man's average caloric intake is higher than a woman's, you may not find yourself losing weight on this plan. In fact, it may contain too many calories for you, and you could end up gaining! Yet the basic principle of the program holds true for women too: If you eat less food, you will lose weight—whether or not you exercise. Should you currently be eating 3,000 or more calories a day (shame on you), this food plan *will* take weight off you. You may not lose as fast as your husband, or as much as you'd like—but it is a sensible, comfortable, and healthy way to trim down.

On this plan you will be feeding your man 1,500 to 2,000 calories daily. If you too want to lose weight, you should adjust the meals or portion sizes for yourself so that you are consuming no more than 1,000 to 1,500 calories per day. I do not think it's healthy to eat less than 1,000 calories a day. (If you insist on eating less than 1,000 calories a day, you must have a physical checkup before beginning the plan and follow it under constant medical supervision.)

But right now, let's get your husband taken care of. In the back of the book, there's a chart for progress. You can write in your own weight, and the weight of everyone else in your family, so that you will be able to see if you too lose weight as your husband surely will. (Use a different color ink for each member of the family.) Remember, even if you are losing weight, your husband will do it faster. *Don't try to keep up with him or be competitive about your progress.* Competition will ruin the fun, and possibly your relationship. This diet is for HIM.

Liberated Does Not Mean Out of the Kitchen

The reason this plan works so well is that your husband—and anyone else you feed—is *fooled* into eating less. This does not happen by magic. It takes hard work. No, let me make that more clear: It takes very, very hard work. And since your husband won't even know what's happening part of the time, the burden of the work falls on you. Just when you thought you were getting liberated, you find yourself back in the kitchen.

Sorry about that. But when you are motivated to save your husband's life, you have to do what you have to do. (Can I have a little violin music, please?)

This food plan allows nights out, restaurant eating, and parties, so don't be discouraged. Its primary focus, however, is at-home cooking, careful food planning, and smart caloric budgeting. If you like to cook, this food plan will make you a happy person. If you don't like being in the kitchen any more than necessary, here's the bad news: To make this weight loss work, you've just *got* to grin and bear it. Both your cooking and shopping styles are going to have to change. You cannot go on the way you have been and expect your husband to lose weight. It'll take time and trouble to adjust to the new cooking style, and it will take perseverance not to fall back to former follies. If it were easy, you would have already done it, right?

Now, the good news:

- Your husband will lose at least twenty pounds (maybe more).
- Your husband will *keep* the weight off.
- The meals you serve will probably be healthier than the ones you normally serve.
- You will be setting a prettier table and making dinner a more festive occasion.
- You'll be making faux-gourmet meals, so they'll be more fun to eat and will impress your family and friends.

If you care enough to buy this book, I know you care enough to pull it off. You are about to begin one of the most rewarding adventures of your life.

2
ADAM'S RIB

Typical Male Excuses

Men say some remarkable things when you ask them why they are overweight. Here's a sampling of some of my husband's responses over the years:

- I'm not overweight, you're just skinny.
- I'm a big guy.
- I can't help it if I have a hearty appetite.
- It's inherited.
- I have big bones.
- Being chunky was my family's way of showing how well off they were—this isn't fat, it's a symbol of success.
- This is protection. I never catch a cold; I haven't been sick in years; I must be doing something right.
- Do you think I'm fat?

All this from a man with an IQ of almost 200!

If you'll look at his statements, you'll note that he either *denies* that he's even got a problem or *rationalizes* that it's *not* beyond his control. He could lose, he thinks, if he set his mind to it. Most revealing was his observation that he has a hearty appetite.

Obviously he does. You don't get to weigh 240 pounds without one. But the underlying message I finally coaxed out of him (why is it that women have to beg their men to verbalize?) was that he considered it unthinkable to stop eating, or to leave the table, when he was still "hungry." (See page 64 Appetite vs. Hunger.)

It was this insight that crystalized my plans. I realized he would never succeed on a weight-loss program that made him feel deprived, that demanded he walk away "hungry," or required he eat "special" foods.

Satisfying his "man-size" appetite is the trick to my plan; in this way, you will be able to se-duce your man into eating less food and losing weight without his knowing. Because he will not be hungry, or at least famished to the point of distraction, he will be on this plan a full two weeks before you admit what's been going on . . . maybe longer. By then, you'll both be happier people.

The Real Reasons Men Eat

Deep down inside, the real reasons men eat, or overeat, are the same as for women. They like food. It makes them feel good. It is their friend. They too experience the stuff-gain-feel-guilty syndrome that women do, yet do not verbalize their concerns as often and do not admit to com-pulsive habits as readily. After all, men are big and strong and like to think they are in control of everything. They would lose respect for them-selves if they thought they were not in control of their bodies, and even when they know they are not, they *act* as if they could lose the weight if they really wanted to.

Women are much quicker to acknowledge that they have a problem, try a self-governing technique, or go for professional help or group support. Men are reluctant to look outside themselves. It generally takes a good bit of prodding to get a man to "go" on a diet or to join a weight-loss group. Although statistics prove that when husbands and wives, or partners, go to class or on a plan together, both parties lose and keep weight off . . . it is women who have to instigate the partnership to get their spouses moving.

Sex and the Fat Cell

Besides the most obvious difference in men's and women's bodies (my five-year-old will be glad to discuss this with you), there are a few differences between the sexes that actually relate to weight loss and to success in a weight-reduction plan.

All men may have been created equal, but women were created more equal: Since their basic mechanical design function is to bear children, their physiology is equipped with a built-in system for gaining weight, storing fat, and bearing and nursing children. As a result, men are free of a burden suffered only by the "weaker" sex. "Women need at least 12 percent body fat just to survive," says Lee Richards, R.N., "with the ideal between 18 and 20 percent. Men need a minimum of 3 percent body fat."

Men stop gaining weight earlier than women.

Male hormones convert calories to muscle where female hormones convert to fat, all be-

34

cause the basic blueprint called for men to be strong and women to be nurturing.

It doesn't take the same amount of willpower for men to lose weight—it's *easier* for them.

Men lose weight almost twice as fast as women do.

With the same amount of exertion, men burn calories almost twice as fast as women.

Male hormones break down fat; female hormones do not.

By the time they are adults, women have twice as much body fat as men.

Men don't take birth control pills, which add hormones that produce fat.

I mention all this not to depress you, but to show you how much easier it's going to be to take weight off your man. You're going to be successful with this plan, you'll feel good about taking the trouble to go through with it, and your husband will have the satisfaction that comes with a victory. If you happen to lose a few pounds along the way, mazel tov. But this plan has been devised specifically for Big Daddy in the hope you can make him less big.

How Fat Is Made

Fat people are not born that way, they are made fat by overeating. Each person, male or female, is born with a set number of fat cells. Before age two and in the years before puberty, if you overeat and store fat, your body develops additional fat cells—which you will feed for the rest of your life. If you do not overeat, you will not gain extra fat cells and you are unlikely to have a weight problem in the future. Once you have those extra fat cells running amok in your body, even if you succeed in taking off excess poundage, you will still have the same inflated number of cells—all calling out for more cheesecake.

Since life is not fair, each person is born with a different number of fat cells, and women are born with more of them than men.

The obvious solution is not to let fat cells be fruitful or multiply. If you have children, you can now do your best to see they never grow up to have a weight problem. Your husband, however, was reared at a time when fat babies were considered healthy babies. His mom didn't know about the perils of excess fat cells. He never had a chance.

If your husband grew up "pudgy," he will never be as svelte as a male model. Remember, his fat cells have *already* been programmed, and it's going to take hard work, love, and patience to beat the clock. Here's the biology lesson his Mom never learned; here's the reason you are now forced to do your stuff to save his life:

Some animal bodies are made for storing fat— seals, birds and bears all have periods when they stuff their faces, but they use up the fat they have stored. Birds fly south for the winter; seals prepare for the mating season and need to be able to outrun those s.o.b.'s with the clubs who are after their pelts; bears hibernate; and so forth. Unfortunately, humans do not have these same automatic mechanisms for chucking off stored fat. When people store fat, they just get fatter—and then sicker and then dead.

This is the way your body works. If you use fewer calories than you eat, your body stores the excess as fat. If you use as many calories as you eat, your body is in balance (thermodynamic balance, to be technical about it) and your weight will remain constant. If you use more calories than you are actually eating, your body will automatically utilize the fat it has already stored for energy. If you run out of stored reserves, your body starts using more vital stores and then you get sick, sick, sick.

Metabolism Blues

"It's my metabolism" has been the war cry of all overweighters since the day Rubens fell out of favor. They envision their metabolism as a little green troll, sitting before a bridge, who won't allow them to pass over to the land of the thin. The bodily process of extracting energy from food is called metabolism, and while some people do have a faster burn-off rate than others, this does not mean metabolism is a set factor that cannot be changed. You can deliberately alter your metabolic rate and thereby lose weight . . . and keep it off. One of the best ways to shift metabolism is through exercise, but it can also be done through new eating patterns that change your setpoint. That's your goal once you begin this plan.

Setpoint

Setpoint refers to the theory that each body works much like a thermostat and that your body can be tuned to, or set, at a certain number that determines how much fat you carry and how many calories you need to eat comfortably to maintain that fat. If you have a high setpoint, you are probably overweight.

The good news: You can readjust your setpoint with hard work and diligence.

Setpoint is defined as precisely the weight you maintain when you are eating normally—not dieting or binging. Thus, when my husband took the Stress Test at a Burbank, California, hospital, it reported that he needed some 3,000 calories to maintain his weight, thus declaring his current setpoint. When you don't eat the amount your body is used to, when you don't live up to your setpoint's expectations, your body feels the change and reacts accordingly, sending mental signals that spell h-u-n-g-e-r.

In order for your husband's weight loss (or yours, for that matter) to be a lifetime change, you must endeavor to change his setpoint to match the new weight goal. This is not as hard as it sounds, because your husband will probably find a new setpoint for himself. Once he has done that, you can pat yourself on the back and relax a little.

Here's what happened to us. We were rolling along, singing a song, and Mike was losing weight automatically. He still took pride in announcing his weight to me every other day or so, but the novelty of the whole thing was beginning to wear off. After about three weeks of silence, I mentioned that I hadn't heard the Weight Report.

"I'm stuck on a plateau," he reported glumly.

Men have picked up this diet phrase without really knowing what it means. You are "stuck on a plateau" when for several days or weeks you cannot seem to lose till suddenly, without explanation, your body shifts back into gear and you continue to drop weight. This phenomenon is more common in women who plateau automatically due to monthly hormonal changes. Either way, you only have a true plateau when you are using the same weight loss techniques as before. It is *not* a plateau if you are eating more and therefore not losing.

I began to watch his form. He had slipped. Not much, mind you, just a tad. But after watching him for three days, I saw he had found a comfortable daily routine that allowed him to eat a lot of food without gaining any weight. *But* he was no longer eating the 1,000 calories a day less that I had prescribed. His body had found an automatic setpoint.

When his weight didn't budge for another two weeks, I suggested that he put himself in my hands for a two-week siege and that I could get him below 200. I thought one big push for God, Queen, country, and goal would make him feel terrific. Instead, he chose not to do anything. He stopped talking about "when I break 200," and seemed to forget he was on any kind of food plan at all. He had found a happy setpoint.

The Ages of Man

There is little difference in the way boys' bodies and girls' bodies assimilate calories until puberty. Then Mother Nature steps in and begins what she has been programmed to do for thousands of years—turn little girls into women and boys into men. As a result, girls stop growing at about age sixteen, yet boys keep on until they are about eighteen. You know how it is: All the girls are taller than all the boys, then suddenly the boys come back to school after a summer at computer camp and discover they are taller than the girls. Oh sure, there will always be tall women, but for the most part, by the time they are eighteen, the boys will have lost their baby fat and have grown to the same height as their fathers. Girls who have not lost their baby fat by the time they are sixteen are not automatically going to lose it. And they are unlikely to be as tall as their fathers.

Men's bodies are in peak condition during the teen years and the early twenties. Ask the army why they like their recruits from eighteen to twenty-one and not from thirty-five to thirty-eight. The body will be its leanest, meanest, and strongest. The twenties are a period of perfection in men's bodies.

In their thirties, men accumulate adipose fat in the trunk and develop what is euphemistically called "middle-age spread." (Women do not suffer from middle-age spread until they are in their forties or fifties!)

To judge whether your man has "middle-age spread" or is merely pudgy, take a good look at his naked body. If he has heavy arms and the fat is fairly well distributed all over his body—he's obese. If the flab is centered on the trunk—it's middle-age spread. Middle-age spread is slightly easier to control because it does not indicate a lifelong trend toward overeating or bad eating habits.

My Husband's Body

Actually, I would like to say that my husband's body is none of your business. But that's not

40

really the case. Because if your husband's body is anything like my husband's, then you too have a problem.

My husband is built like his parents, which is to be expected. He is not as heavy as Buddha or Santa Claus, nor as slim as Abraham Lincoln or Ichabod Crane. Genetically speaking, he could *never* look like Lincoln or Crane. But still, he could look like a thinner version of his parents and be a lot healthier!

Before Diet

Before he lost the weight, my husband's body was a little bit more than pudgy. In clothes (okay, the size 42's I insisted he buy were too big, but the 40's were too tight . . .), he merely appeared "big" with maybe a spare tire or two fitting smoothly into his extra-large shirts. Naked, well, that was another story:

- Lying on his side, he looked about the way I did just before our baby was born.
- Sitting up, with his shoulders and back rounded, he had breasts!
- Standing, he had two or three distinct rolls, and I don't mean of the Royce variety. These are familiarly referred to as "love handles."

After Diet

- Flat tummy in clothes or out
- Flat chest
- Only one love handle

People who lose a lot of weight are often unhappy with their new bodies because of all the sag and bag. When a man loses about twenty

41

pounds, only his belly diminishes because this is where the adipose fat is lodged. When he loses more than that, his chest begins to subside as well. That's when he needs exercise. If you can lead your husband to fitness, congratulations! But just remember this: My husband lost his weight without exercise, kept the weight off without it, and has not had a jiggle problem.

Check out your husband tonight and see if there's room for improvement. Unsightly flab should be a warning sign it's time for you to take over and get him back to size.

Cultural Overeating

In my studies of my husband's eating patterns, I've noticed a few distinct problems that have to do with his maleness or my *interpretation* of his maleness:

• I give him larger portions of food than anyone else at the table—even when we have company and there are other men present. He is bigger, stronger, hungrier, and all those quintessentially macho things. Breadwinners are supposed to be bread eaters, or something like that.

• I give him my unfinished foods. I know it's a sin to waste food, so I never throw out a leftover . . . I give it to my husband, the omnivore. If I can only eat half of the banana, I never force myself to finish it, but give it to my husband, who quickly makes "all gone." He performs the exact same function for our son (the type who takes one bite, then says he's finished).

• I cater to his food needs because he's the king of the castle. Even independent women make sure the cabinets are stocked with their husbands' favorite foods. They usually *serve* them too. While I am not a slave who waits on any man, if I am going downstairs to the kitchen to get a pen out of my purse, I ask Mike if he wants anything. "Yeah," he says, "maybe an ice cream sandwich." I go downstairs (using a few calories), I get my pen and the ice cream sandwich and then go upstairs, using a few more calories. I have nothing to eat and have burned some calories and exercised my leg muscles. He's been lying on the bed reading a spy yarn and is about to eat 103 more calories. (Weight Watchers ice cream sandwiches have 103 calories.) If he's having the guys over for the monthly poker game, I wouldn't think of not having food and beer in the house and virtually laying it at their feet . . . this is my notion of what the hostess should do—even if it means killing the guests with kindness and calories.

There has been some research recently on the secret eating patterns of women—women who eat small-to-moderate meals in family and social situations and then, in private, binge on any number of outlandish foods, all representing warmth, comfort, love, reassurance, or whatever is needed that day. This is primarily a female syndrome, probably because men don't have to be shy about it. Society respects those "hearty" appetites; we stuff our men in front of everyone and condone their overeating as a masculine virtue. And then we cry at their funerals.

Why Men Can Keep It Off Once They Lose It

According to Dr. Maria Simonson, once men have lost weight they tend to keep it off. Women *worry* more about their weight and know more about calories. But they are also more likely to fall prey to crash diets and crazy schemes that promise fast, but not long-term, weight loss.

Men are more successful because:

- The weight loss process was satisfying. Because a man can eat so much food and keep his weight steady, he usually does not feel deprived and therefore lives a comfortable and lighter life-style. Maintenance for a woman is often such a difficult task, she can't help but splurge or relax herself into the next size.
- Men get positive feedback from being thinner. Women like to look "good" for certain events, then tend to let themselves go, and gain weight back. Men lose to lose.
- Male body composition is in their favor.
- Men who add exercise and/or sports to their life-style are more likely to stick to an exercise program than women are. Many men work for companies that pay them to exercise.
- Doctors report that of their patients who lose twenty or more pounds, men have a better chance of keeping the weight off than women.

Shocking News

I read an unnamed survey in *The Health and Fitness Handbook* that announced these shocking figures:

- *Only* 50 percent of the overweight women surveyed realized they were overweight.
- *Only* 25 percent of the overweight men realized they were overweight.

• *Only* 10 percent of those surveyed were planning to reduce.

I don't know if this means that women have better eyesight than men, but it is a dramatic commentary on why your husband is overweight.

You *can* help yourself to live healthier and longer by making changes in diet and life-style. And when you do it with a partner, you have a greater chance for success. A 1975 study at Brown University showed that dieters with partners (most frequently husband- and wife-teams) lost up to three times as much weight as a control group of solo dieters—and maintained the weight loss over a two-year follow-up period.

Operation Observation

Before you begin this plan, spend a few days observing your husband's eating habits, food intake, and snack techniques. Note how much he eats, how often he eats, and why you think he's eating. In my assessment of Mike, I discovered:

• He has very bad table habits, probably learned in childhood. This is not to say that he doesn't put his napkin in his lap, but I've seen him stand behind his chair and serve his plate before he sits down. He reaches across the table without asking for something to be passed. He'll read the paper while eating breakfast, unless I tell him it's tacky. He'll not only clean his plate but will finish off any one- or two-bite leftovers that are on the serving platters. He eats fast and always wants more.

• He snacks twice a day—a 10:00 A.M. coffee break and a bedtime treat.

• He doesn't understand enough about nutrition and calories to see that he consistently chooses the wrong foods while patting himself on the back for watching his weight. For example, he'll order a chef's salad in a restaurant rather than an entrée (a nice start, but . . .), then he hits the bread basket, eats the whole salad, and tops it off with *blue cheese* dressing. (Blue cheese has a high percent of fat and should be avoided!) I promise you, he has not saved one calorie nor done his body one bit of good with this meal. But he thinks that he's been a martyr to his health.

• He thinks highly caloric treats are "owed" him when he's had either an especially bad or a very good day. I suspect that to jazz up ordinary or boring days he also thinks he's entitled to a "treat."

• He associates food with happy times and with his happy childhood. Say we're having a dull evening at home, there's nothing to watch on TV, and a change of pace would liven things up. "Let's all go to Howard Johnson's for an ice cream soda," he says. Having an ice cream soda is an old family treat for him (it was a tradition during my childhood too), so not only are we getting out of the house and relieving our boredom, but we are taking our parents and our happy memories along.

Once you see how and when someone is overeating, you can start to look at the why's. Perhaps some of the reasons are too deep for you to tackle. Never mind, save those for later. This food plan will still work. If you are observant, you'll get a good understanding of his eating patterns, which will help provide a happy day of eating, but with fewer calories.

If you need assistance "observing" during office hours, enlist a little help—does he have a secretary or office chum? A woman will be a better help to you than a man, and for heaven's sake, don't make it look like you're asking her to spy. ("Gee, Jennifer, I'm working on this project for my husband, but I *really* need your help to make it work . . .")

Keep track of his meals and nibbles for a few days:

Breakfast:	
Coffee Break:	
Lunch:	
Coffee Break:	
Cocktails:	
Dinner:	
Snacks:	

chapter **3**

ALIMENTARY,
MY DEAR EVE

Why Fad Diets Will Not Work

There will always be fad diets because they offer the American dream—instant, easy results. But thinking people know, deep down inside, that fad diets *never* work. Sure, you may take ten pounds off quickly—but you'll gain it back. You'll suffer from the yo-yo syndrome and you'll have a closet with two wardrobes, your "fat" clothes and your "thin" clothes. In the end, you'll mostly be frustrated, angry, sick, and heavy.

Anyone with a strong sense of willpower can follow a strict food plan for ten to fourteen days and take off ten pounds. But those plans are not safe for everyday living and do not offer the ease or comfort we have come to demand from our regular meals. They always stand for deprivation. They are programs to be "on" until you go "off" them—they are not life-style plans. The only successful diet doesn't *feel* like a diet.

48

Why This Plan Works

This weight loss plan works because it demands *few* changes from your husband—or any other person on it who is trying to slim down. In fact, I find the diet harder for the person doing the cooking than for the person doing the losing. (But that's only my opinion, and it's based on the fact that I hate to cook.)

Look at it this way, any plan that can be implemented without your husband's knowing it, can't be so difficult that he will be miserable. If he's not miserable, he won't go off the diet. In fact, part of the time, he won't know he's on it. Your husband's life will improve when he is on this food plan, and that is why it will work.

The Sneaky Approach

I do not advocate keeping secrets from one's spouse.

Usually.

I have never lied to my husband, or withheld important information. I confessed about splurging at that shoe sale at Joseph's as soon as I walked in the door; I have never considered hiding the American Express bill. I have a tell-all personality to begin with: I can't keep a secret worth a damn and am crummy at surprises. *However*, I admit that I used the Sneaky Approach on my husband for the first two weeks of this plan— and I might have gone even longer had not ego, pure and simple (mine, not his), stepped in the way.

You do not have to follow in my footsteps. You can tell your husband your plans, even discuss them with him, or read this book together. But in *my* case, for *my* husband, I *knew* that being sneaky was the only way to make this work. Here's why:

- I definitely thought the ends justified the means.
- I clearly remember my mother saying that sometimes it's kinder to tell a white lie than to tell the truth. I'm very big on kindness.
- I think that there are some things you talk about and some things you just *do*.
- I wasn't at all sure Mike would cooperate if I laid my cards on the kitchen table. (He'd been violently opposed to other weight loss methods and I had no hope that he might have changed his mind.)
- I thought we'd both have something to be proud of when we had some results, and nothing to motivate us until there *was* progress.
- I wanted to see if I could pull it off.

The Sneaky Approach will only work until your husband's pants fall down; after that you'll probably be forced to admit what you're up to unless you are either very coy or your husband is very slow.

(I'll never forget the night, exactly two weeks after I began this plan, when my husband very casually said, "You know, honey, I must be doing something right, my pants are too big." I mean, really!)

You may opt for Sneaky and find that (a) you get caught early on and have to confess, or (b) your husband *never* catches on and you can go Sneaky all the way. If you don't want to be sneaky, that's fine with me. If you want to be *really sneaky,* take the jacket off this book and replace it with one from a Jackie Collins novel.

The Upfront Approach

If you decide to play it straight, you know best how to deal with your husband.

Leaving this book lying around will probably take care of the whole problem.

The Back Door Approach

If you are unable to go Sneaky but feel that Upfront won't work for you, try what I call the Back Door Approach. Announce you are going on a new food plan for yourself. After he begins to lose weight on "your" plan, talk about his full cooperation.

Where to Start

Since this program is essentially in your hands, and I'm assuming you've gone the Sneaky or Back Door route, you can begin the plan any time you like. I suggest, however, that you not start within two weeks of a vacation or a holiday. Please give yourself, and your husband, every opportunity to achieve a victory. The best time is today—an ordinary day in your regular life. Give yourself two or three days to prepare, then commence. (The preparation is mostly observation and grocery shopping, combined with a little kitchen cleanup—you don't have to be cooking or memorizing food charts for three days.)

Start without fanfare; make as few pronouncements as possible. This is a time for action, not words. The steps are very simple: operation observation, kitchen cleanup, new grocery shopping, and it's *faux* gourmet all the way. The recipes at the back of the book will help you get started or you can experiment on your own.

Less Is More

This food plan has no gimmicky name or cutesy handle for you to remember it by because it's neither trick nor fad. It's safe, it's doctor-approved, and it works. It operates on one basic principle:

LESS IS MORE

When a person eats less food, he or she will automatically lose weight. This is a simple fact. For most men, because they can eat as many as 2,000 calories a day and still lose weight, eating less is merely a matter of your manipulating the ingredients on the plate.

It will not hurt anyone in your family to eat less —except for active teens and athletes in training. There is no question your husband will notice some sort of change, but chances are good he won't notice exactly *what* the difference is. More than likely, the 1,000 calories a day you will be taking away from him were usually lost in so-called "empty" calories and will not be sorely missed.

You will be using a method of vague calorie counting I call *calorie budgeting*. It works exactly like your family financial budget. Your man is allowed 1,500 to 2,000 calories a day. You must do this on a daily, not a weekly, basis, so he doesn't overeat one day and fast the next. You will be serving him (or seeing that he eats) three meals a day; I do not recommend skipping meals. Let me make that a bit stronger: I am violently opposed to anyone skipping meals. Each meal is budgeted at approximately 500 calories; you then have another 500 to play around with in the form of desserts, snacks, drinks, mathematical mistakes, or whatever. After all, you will not be counting, just estimating; the leeway frees you from carrying a calculator or keeping large sums scribbled on your memory. (To get familiar with calorie counts, check the calorie section of the book, page 171.)

For every 3,500 calories a person eats and does not burn off, a pound is gained. You can lose weight by burning more calories (exercise) or by consuming fewer calories. (Less *is* more.) It takes a good bit of exercise to work off a pound (jumping rope for seven hours!), and many people prefer to eat less food to control their weight.

My plan *tricks* a man into eating less food and renders us triumphant. Eve was on the right track when she reached for that apple if she wanted it for Adam's dinner. . . .

A 1,000 calorie diet (the kind most women are forced to submit to) is pretty tight and requires extreme discipline; but a 2,000 calorie diet is not much of a hardship. If your man does not lose weight on 2,000 calories a day, you can cut him back by another 500 calories. Or, if he is really a nosher, you may want to reduce his calories gradually: Cut him back to 2,500 a day for a while and then cut back another 500 a few weeks later.

According to Dr. Alan R. Marston, you will lose weight automatically (and without exercise) at these caloric intakes:

Men	1,500 calories
Women weighing over 200 pounds	1,500 calories
Women weighing 130–200 pounds	1,200 calories
Women weighing 130 pounds	1,000 calories

The New Math: Finding the Proper Calorie Count

I first got the idea for this food plan when I accidentally discovered how many calories it took my husband to "maintain" his then current weight of almost 240 pounds. The results of his Stress Test emerged on a multi-paged computer printout that was even more fascinating than a computerized horoscope. I was simultaneously mesmerized and horrified. He was eating over 3,000 calories a day! I had never considered his weight in terms of calories before, nor did I go one step further to realize he could eat well on at least a thousand calories less a day. To me, 3,000 calories was an embarrassment of riches.

You do not need to know your husband's daily calorie intake to implement this diet, but it will show you how many calories you have to play with and will give you a clear-eyed look at his specific problem. If you automatically cut him down by 500 calories a day, he will lose a pound a week; 1,000 calories a day, two pounds a week. Knowing his calorie count will help you set your goal and establish your balancing act, which if you are being Sneaky will help you. (If you reduce by too much, he may notice!) Never attempt to lose more weight by a so-called "faster" method. It's unhealthful.

To get the number of calories needed to maintain weight at its current level (setpoint), choose one of the categories that best fits the amount of physical exercise your husband has in a regular day (not a weekend) and multiply his current weight by the number next to his category on this chart.*

PHYSICAL EXERTION LEVEL	MULTIPLY WEIGHT BY
extremely inactive	13
less active than average	14
reasonably active	15
very active	17
extremely active	21

Using this technique, I would take my husband's old weight 240 and multiply it by 13 to get 3,120! To find the number of calories he should be eating to reach a particular new weight, multiply the *desired* weight by one of the numbers on the chart. If I thought my husband should weigh 200 pounds, his reduced calorie intake would be 200 × 13 = 2,600. That's a 500 calorie difference, approximately, and believe me, 500 calories can be taken out of a daily routine merely by skipping a few drinks or a piece of pie and a bedtime snack.

I did not use the chart method to figure out how many calories to cut out of Mike's diet, but merely threw up my hands in horror and withdrew an arbitrary 1,000 calories from his life. It is

*Chart information from Dr. Kelley Bronwell, University of Pennsylvania.

harder to cut out 1,000 calories than 500 and go undetected, but I wanted results and felt I could handle the gamble. It worked!

- If he eats 500 calories a day less, he will lose one pound a week.
- If he eats 1,000 calories a day less, he will lose two pounds a week.

Finding the Goal

When I put my husband on his food plan, I did not have a specific weight goal in mind. I merely wanted to see a steady loss. Although a doctor or insurance chart would probably say that a man my husband's height (5'11") with his family medical history should weigh 175 to 180 pounds, I long ago realized he could never weigh that little. After the famous liquid protein diet he weighed 185—for a week or two. And he did look handsome and healthy. But he couldn't hold it. Personally, I've always thought that as long as he didn't cross 200 (and if he also did some aerobic exercise), he'd be safe.

I do realize this is on the high side and we must both watch his health carefully, but you can't expect miracles and you can't nag your husband to death, or you will end by outwitting yourself!

Mike set his own goals after he began to lose steadily. He first went for 220; once there, he began to look at 200. When he got to 205, he started talking about 185. I never said a word. (Clearly, this was not easy for me.)

While everyone should have a goal as something to look forward to, the goal should not be too far away. If I had said to my husband,

"Honey, you need to lose fifty pounds," he would have replied, "Honey, I have just put in a call to Marvin Mitchelson."

It is much more encouraging to reach your goal and be forced to set a new one. That's why this book is geared to a twenty-pound weight loss. (If your husband does go for a greater loss, talk him into a medical checkup.) My husband happened to lose thirty-five pounds before he began to "plateau." Your husband may lose even more.

Twenty pounds is something to be proud of—it can make a difference in health, in appearance, and in self-esteem. The day your man walks into a room and someone who has not seen him in a while remarks, "Boy, you've sure lost weight," he will be very, very happy.

One of the worst traps you can fall prey to is to set a mental goal for your husband and push him toward it. This food plan takes a lot of your time and patience. You can get so involved in it that you personally want to assault each pound. It's easy to think you are managing a race horse; don't get carried away in order to satisfy your own competitive spirit.

Body Type, Insurance Charts, and Weight Scales

My husband is an endomorph—one of God's pear-shaped people. Endomorphs are built to be a little bit shorter, a little bit rounder, and a little bit stockier than everybody else.

I am an ectomorph, the tall, thin, angular type who has trouble gaining weight. I have been called Olive Oyl all of my life and have been on serious weight gain plans since I was twelve.

The average body type is called the meso-morph—he or she has the best chance of keeping weight stable and is the most athletically built of the three basic types, though in no way guaranteed to be perfect.

When you begin to calculate your husband's potential weight loss and his goal weight, it is important to take body type into consideration. Endomorphs should be allowed to remain stocky (without being sloppy, of course), since you can never change their basic build. If the weight chart you happen to use has only one suggested weight for your husband's height, consider that weight to be proper for mesomorphs. Allow five pounds over for endomorphs and five pounds under for ectomorphs. If you're married to an overweight ectomorph (very rare!), congratulations, we're going to give you a free five pounds —if you want them.

Insurance charts and weight scales are curious creatures in that not only can you find variations on them, but you can find contradictions as well. In recent years, some experts have announced that the optimal weights listed on weight charts are too low!

Most doctors will give their patients a ten-pound range within which they are free to find their ideal weight. I've also heard of the mirror test which is simple enough—you stand in front of a full-length mirror, naked, and take a cold, hard look at yourself. If you are cosmetically overweight, you need to lose weight. (This test does not work for anorectics, please note, because no matter what they weigh, they still think they are fat. But I must assume you would not have bought this book if your man was anorectic! Besides, most anorectics are women.)

If the naked truth doesn't do it for you, try this method: Allow 110 pounds for the first five feet of your husband's height, then add five pounds for each additional inch. Add ten pounds for a large frame; subtract ten pounds for a small frame.

If you do not know how much your husband should weigh, even approximately, call his doctor and ask.

Breaking Bad Habits

In your analysis of your husband's eating patterns, you will probably observe several bad habits that foster his hand-to-mouth coordination. In order for him to lose weight and keep it off, he is going to have to conquer them. Breaking habits is never easy, especially ones that have lingered since childhood. Luckily for men, however, it is a bit easier for them to be programmed because they are used to being taken care of at meal time.

The person who does the food preparation and presentation will always have a harder time adjusting to new food habits because he or she is surrounded by food.

To help him break his pattern, you have to practice diplomacy. *Don't demand changes, just make changes for him,* but make the changes *wonderful.* Ease him into the new life-style, and make it *better* than the old.

Here is a list of common bad habits leading to weight gain. It's unusual for just one member of a family to have all these habits; probably you are as guilty as your husband. If it's hard to spot the problems, invite a friend or thin family member to observe your meals and eating patterns.

Bad Habit #1: *Skipping Meals*

People who are watching their weight often falsely assume that by skipping a meal they have automatically sealed in a calorie loss. This is rarely true because he or she will eat twice as much at lunch, or will have a sweet coffee break in search of a pick-me-up. Skipping meals is one of the worst ways in the world to lose weight.

While breakfast need not be elaborate, you should have some kind of meal and eat it *sitting* at the table. (See Bad Habit #3.) I'm an advocate of a big breakfast because most of it will be burned off during the day. Besides, it appeals to a man's sense of macho (big men start their big days with a big meal . . .).

Men who are salesmen or who work alone are often tempted to skip lunch because either they don't like to take the time for the break or they don't like to eat alone. A man who drives a territory is often tempted to grab a snack to eat while driving, instead of eating a real meal that he would have to consume alone. Men who have no one to lunch with are often tempted to skip lunch altogether and snack through the afternoon instead.

Once your man knows about this food plan, he will learn to appreciate lunch more. In fact, he'll soon learn that it is his best opportunity to cheat a little. Since it's unlikely that it will be possible for you to be with your man at lunchtime, you're just going to have to shrug your shoulders and pretend to be relaxed. It is better for a person to overeat at lunch than to skip it!

As for skipping dinner, I've never known a man who considered such a crazy idea.

Bad Habit #2: *Eating at Odd Hours*

I don't want to ruin the free-flowing momentum of your life, or pin you down to restrictions of time and place, but people who don't eat regular meals at regular times usually end up gaining weight. Even if you are one of those who believes in six mini-meals a day, all six should be at a specific time and a specific number of hours apart. If you eat all day long, you will get fat. Honest.

For men who work from nine to five, or thereabouts, the structuring of meals is relatively easy —breakfast must be eaten before they leave for the office, lunch is sometime between twelve and two, and dinner is after they get home from work. So far so good. Men under pressure begin by skipping meals and end up eating all day: They have lunch sent up by a fast-food restaurant that delivers at 3:00 P.M. ("I had a bear of a day, honey! I didn't even get to grab a bite of lunch until after three!") Then they go home to dinner three hours later, having performed no exercise —save leaving the office and climbing into the car—for the entire day. Breakfast should be four to five hours before lunch, dinner should be at least five hours later. The only excuses I'll accept are from those crossing time zones on an airplane.

Men who work night shifts, who stay up twenty-four hours at a clip, or who work indoors where you can't tell day from night have a more difficult time. They must be forced to eat at regular intervals and to ignore the availability of nosh foods.

Bad Habit #3: *Eating Away From the Table*

You'd be surprised how many Americans don't eat at their tables. They get really creative—eating in cars, in offices, in front of television sets, climbing into bed with a tray. Maybe they think variety is the spice of life. The fact is that if you are doing something else while you are eating, you are not concentrating on your food and therefore will not keep track of what or how much you are eating. When the Dodgers are losing, my husband is capable of eating everything we have in the house, and then asking what's for dinner. If our son is eating while watching TV he will only want the foods he sees advertised—usually the sugar-coated variety. This is human nature and must be combated by limiting the places where you take your meals. Eat all three meals *at the table*. Never eat while you are working or doing something else. Never eat standing up or lying down. If you take your lunch to work with you, get out of the office to eat it whenever possible.

Bad Habit #4: *Serving Family Style*

Family-style eating—in which all the food is put in serving dishes on the table so that people can help themselves—is a very nice idea. I happen to have invested a lot of money in the serving pieces that go with my china and I feel terrible whenever I realize that I am not using them. But in a family of overeaters, serving family style is a serious mistake because it encourages people to eat more than they should.

To control calorie intake you must be able to control the size of the portions. You can't sit at the head of the table with a whip in your hand, so you might as well eliminate temptation. Put the portions on the plates in the kitchen. Calculate the meal so that there are no leftovers. This makes the cleanup easier and keeps waistlines trim.

Bad Habit #5: *Using Food for Comfort or Reward*

The first day my son stayed at school until three in the afternoon, he had to take lunch with him. Since I wanted this to be a wonderful experience and to reinforce how great it was to stay all day, I prepared him his favorite lunch. Not only did I run out to the fast-food chicken store for the precise part of the chicken's anatomy he prefers, but I drove another mile and a half to a bakery where they make the kind of chocolate cupcakes he likes. I also threw in a small package of Doritos, one of those cute packages of fruit juice, and a napkin with Snoopy on it.

Let's look at what I did. First of all, the nutritional value of that meal stinks. Second, I wasted a lot of time, trouble, and money. But worst of all, I sent out a psychological message that said, "If you stay at school until three, you will be rewarded with *food*." (I stood in the corner and punished myself when I realized what I had done.)

Your mother-in-law did the same thing to your husband. And many other things much worse. She kissed his booboos and made them better with a brownie. She soothed hurt feelings with home-baked cookies. She made Christmas and Chanukah and Easter and Halloween and birthdays special with her sugar-coated treats sealed not only with her tasty message of love, but with the underlying notion that *food makes everything better.*

If you are an adult and still think this way, you probably have a weight problem. It will take a lot of work to convince yourself (or your man) that food is merely a nice way to keep the machinery operating.

Bad Habit #6: *Snacking*

Snacking was created by boredom and serves not only to break the monotony of the job you are doing, but to comfort or reward you (see above) for having done any work at all. It is a psychological habit just like smoking. In order to give yourself permission to stop work, you have to have something else to do; therefore, you smoke a cigarette, or eat a little snack.

If your husband is a snacker, find out why he is eating and try to solve that problem. While there are social occasions requiring you to eat between meals, you should not be hungry then and you should be able to say no politely or merely to nibble. My husband was eating over 500 calories a day in snacks! For many, just eliminating this extra amount of food (or drink!) can bring on a substantial weight loss.

Appetite vs. Hunger

While you don't have to go to a Third World nation to see hunger, most overweight Americans suffer from a problem with appetite, not hunger.

There is a crucial difference. You will need to learn this difference and later on, your husband must learn it:

Hunger is a biological state in which your body *requires* food to keep on going.

Appetite is a psychological state in which you *think* that you are hungry and end up eating to satisfy your mind, not your body.

Appetite can be developed over a period of time, or can be associated with specific events. Work avoidance often triggers appetite.

Those so-called hunger pangs that you give in to are regular stomach contractions that occur whether you are fasting or eating. These contractions are normal and mean absolutely nothing. (My doctor promised.) You have been falsely taught that this contraction means "hunger," so your mind allows you to eat even when your body isn't hungry. The stomach can stretch to accommodate a large meal, yet it always returns to its regular size. The ability to stretch is instigated by the psychological response that tells you to keep putting food into your mouth.

After my husband had lost his first ten pounds on my plan, and we had gone through exactly two weeks of trick and treat, I explained to him the difference between hunger and appetite. I had tried this before, but he never listened. It was about 10:00 P.M., and he was getting out of bed to make his ritual trip to the kitchen. I asked him to skip the snack tonight. He got angry. Then I sprang the *big news*, explaining that he hadn't lost that ten pounds by accident, that I had been working creatively to make it happen and since he had come so far without helping me, he could get even farther if he pitched in. His job was to

65

stop snacking and to bear "hunger" with the new understanding that it was merely appetite. An unfulfilled appetite will subside as the eating habit is broken. The next two weeks without his bedtime snack were hard for him, and he did feel deprived. He felt *deprived*, he didn't feel hungry. After that he adjusted and stopped talking about it. When he reached his "plateau" period, I noticed he was eating an apple at night.

Emotional Satisfaction

The trick to this plan is to give your husband the emotional satisfaction he seeks from food in a reduced-calorie diet or through some other method. (Sex?) When I discovered how important the bedtime apple was to my husband, I adjusted his calorie budget to allow him 100 calories at night time. Haven't you always found that the key to satisfying a man is being flexible?

4

LESS IS MORE

The First Two Weeks

The first two weeks of this diet are the hardest—
for you, not him. You are:

- going it alone, since he doesn't even know
  what's happening;
- adjusting to a new type of cooking;
- forced into a few white lies that may keep you
  walking a tightrope;
- wondering if you're going to see results, or if
  you will have gone through all this for nothing.

But there's also something very exciting about
this period. You have a special secret (not as exciting as a love affair but much safer and you'll
be caught up in the game like nature of the challenge. This is something special only you can do,
and if you tackle it with zest, you'll find your
enthusiasm will carry you over the tight spots.

For your husband, the first two weeks will be
the easiest, although he may look back at them
and think you behaved a little oddly. He may
wonder about the sudden shift in food, the sudden home improvements, and why the table is

looking more elegant. Playing dumb will get you through these awkward moments.

You will find that the two weeks will pass quickly, and your husband will shed pounds. If, at the end of two weeks, he hasn't said anything, you can keep on being sneaky. If you don't have a bathroom scale, now is the time to buy one, so you can get him to weigh in (just like Garfield) and discover his happy surprise. If he doesn't happen to notice he's lost weight, don't get upset. Just keep plugging away. He *will* eventually.

Breaking the News

Since each marriage is different, each wife has to decide on her own when to tell her man what she's been up to. I suggest you go as long as you can *without* telling him, simply because he'll be happier. And what's a woman's lot but to suffer in silence?

In my case, I just couldn't keep my mouth shut while he kept marveling about this mysterious transformation, and when an opportune moment came my way, I went directly into my rap about appetite and hunger.

It was difficult to explain to my husband what I'd done without belittling him or making myself sound too grand. I really wanted him to know how hard the two weeks had been for me, how much extra time it took, and how dedicated a wife I must be to have done this. But if you lay it on too heavy, he'll announce that he never asked you to go through all this in the first place and that his weight is his problem, not yours. Tread carefully!

If he gets suspicious and *asks* you what's going

on while you're still in your *sneaky* mode, tell him

- it's just some wild and wacky idea you'd like to give a try;
- *he* gave you the idea;
- you're trying to lose weight and would appreciate his going along with your new food plan for a few weeks;
- you just wanted to show him how much you love him, and how much you want him to be around over the next fifty years.

When you *are* ready to tell him what's going on in a serious way, underline your love and concern rather than your ability to manipulate his diet or control his life. Don't make yourself sound long-suffering or martyred; don't dump on his weight problem. Act as if the diet is a bouquet of flowers you are giving him because you care.

Calorie Budgeting

Some people are compulsive eaters. I am a compulsive shopper. So I know from budgeting. Each month I allow myself a certain amount of money for clothes. That's it. I have to spend it in cash and when it's gone, the party's over—until the next month. Calorie budgeting works precisely the same way, except rather than a monthly plan, it is a *daily* exercise.

Just as you figure out what clothes you can purchase over the month to roughly equal your budget—without going into debt or losing the house—you will be loosely managing calories so that by the time your husband goes to sleep each night, you will have credited his account with

69

2,000 calories. (More or less—you will arrive at your precise calorie budget based on the mathematical calculations that you did. See page 55.)

Try to spend the calories in the basic food groups (see page 85), making sure his meals are low-cal but also nutritious and as devoid of "empty" calories as possible. While this diet is not a high-fiber diet, make sure you balance fiber into your budget. (See page 107.)

To give you an example of how calorie budgeting works, here are two dinners that could have been served on any night at my home—*before* the sneak diet:

DINNER #1

1 porterhouse steak per person, approximately
16 ounces with bone, yielding approximately
     8 ounces of meat
    Large baked potato with sour cream and
      cheddar cheese and butter
    Frozen string beans with butter or margarine
    Salad (with packaged salad dressing)
    Tea or coffee
    No dessert

DINNER #2

2 boned and skinned chicken breasts stuffed
    with chopped mushrooms, zucchini and
    mozzarella cheese (two per person)
    Brown rice
    Salad with packaged salad dressing
    Tea or coffee
    No dessert

The calorie count on Dinner #1 is slightly over 1,400; Dinner #2 is about 700. Incredible difference for two very similar meals, isn't it? My husband could probably lose weight by cutting out snacks and eating dinners like #2. Or I could refine Dinner #2 slightly, reducing it by 100 to 150 calories.

Empty Calories

There are two types of calories that are so sneaky you hardly realize you are eating them: hidden calories and empty calories. Hidden calories are the ones that are in regular, everyday foods—but you don't suspect they are there, unless you are sophisticated at calorie-counting. A steak has more calories than the average eater would ever guess. Look at Dinner #1 and Dinner #2, and see the difference those hidden calories can make.

Empty calories, which are usually not well hidden, offer little or no nutrition for their caloric content. For example, a tablespoon of peanut butter may have about 100 calories, but it's a great food—it's tasty, has little or no cholesterol, is high in nutrients, and isn't expensive. A piece of candy may have the same 100 calories, but it offers your body nothing but sugar. *Those* are empty calories. Most junk foods consist of empty calories, which is why eliminating them can make such a dramatic impact on your waistline. Liquor consists of empty calories; most desserts are filled with empty calories.

When you are counting calories, you do not have the budget to waste anything. To make your calories go as far as they can, eliminate as many *empty* calories as possible. Allow yourself (or your man) no more than 100 calories a day for liquor (if he drinks); 100 for a snack (if snacks cannot be eliminated); and 150 for dessert—I don't think desserts should be eliminated.

Look for hidden calories in these foods:

- fruits
- fruit juices
- meats

Look for empty calories in these foods:

- candies and sweets
- chips, pretzels, etcetera
- desserts
- sauces, dressings, and toppings
- refined-flour products
- packaged meats
- soft drinks

The Well-Rounded Diminished Diet

Once you start talking about "refining" menus and cutting back the amount of food you serve, make sure you are providing the nutrients the body needs. Eliminate junk whenever possible. Serve a meal that is low in fats, sugars, and salt and that, instead, is high in fiber, protein, fruit, and vegetables—not additives or condiments. While many people are advocates of eating something from each of the four food groups, you may end up with too fatty a diet that way and with insufficient fiber. I suggest you think of the balanced meal as composed of three elements: One Fruits & Vegetables selection, plus one Animal

Foods & Nuts selection, plus one Pasta & Staples selection equals a very nice meal.

FRUITS & VEGETABLES	ANIMAL FOODS & NUTS	PASTA & STAPLES
citrus fruits	beans and lentils	pasta
green vegetables	cheese	potato
root vegetables	eggs	rice
soft fruits and	nuts	bread
berries	meat	cereal
apples, pears, etc.	poultry	
	fish	
	milk	

I've made my calories go as far as they can by using this method. It is essential that you not buy too many shoes with your calories, or too many little black dresses—the well-rounded diet, like the well-rounded wardrobe, needs a little of everything.

Size Does Count

There is no denying the relationship between calorie intake and portion size. No matter what the number of calories in any one item, the more you eat, the more calories you consume. The *Less Is More* plan

1. cuts down the size of the portions and therefore eliminates a good number of the calories consumed;
2. cuts out empty calories.

What you're really doing is an intricate juggling act: decreasing the portion size of high-calorie foods and increasing the portion size of low-calorie foods so that you can reduce total caloric consumption by about 1,000 per day without changing the basic structure of your meal.

- You will often be serving less food on the plate.
- You will be serving more of some foods than others.
- You will not be cutting out certain foods just because they are "fattening"; instead, you will serve them less frequently and in smaller-sized portions.

I am convinced that one of the reasons men eat so much is that they are served more than anyone else in the family. Or they get used to eating a lot when they are active, growing, teenage boys and neglect to taper down when their bodies mature. Whatever the reason, if your man is consuming more than 2,000 calories a day, he can cut back to that number without suffering—physically or emotionally. (Unless he is a marathon runner.)

Since I do not believe in strict calorie counting, or in measuring or weighing food, you are going to have to practice a little bit to discover the right size portion for your husband's new food plan. If I were putting you (or your man) on a strict, old-fashioned diet, I would say that for dinner you are allowed a 4- to 6-ounce piece of chicken breast. On my food plan, I do not weigh anything or ask you to weigh anything. You merely choose either the largest, plumpest breast from the package of skinless, boneless breasts, or the two smallest; then pound the one large breast or the two small breasts together into the largest possible shape, so that it looks like a lot of food. We all know how deceiving looks can be.

The size of a portion of fruit, vegetable, pasta, or filler should generally be about the size of a scoop of ice cream. You will learn to fill out the plate by the arrangement of the food or by filling in with less fattening tidbits—increase the amount of vegetables; decrease the size of the "main entrée."

Familiarize yourself with standard calorie counts by consulting the Calorie Counts chart (see page 171). Note specifically the items you fix often. If I don't mention one of your brands or a favorite food, get the count off the box or the label. The idea is not to memorize scads of numbers, but to know offhand that almost any one-ounce piece of cheese costs 100 calories; that almost any cut of beef, pork, or lamb costs 100 calories per ounce, etcetera. Just as you are familiar with food prices, you need to become familiar with calorie costs. Then you can round them out in your head as you prepare a meal. You may want to buy a calorie-counter book to keep around the house, in the kitchen, or at your desk. There are several guides available in book stores; I often use *Le Gette's Calorie Encyclopedia* and keep it on my desk in the office. Whenever I want to take a break, or need a divertissement while my nail polish is drying, I leaf through it. I find it fascinating reading, and I always learn something new.

The Sort-of-Taboo List

One of the worst things about many conventional diets is the list of things you shouldn't eat. The list includes everything worth living for; the dieter becomes so discouraged he doesn't even want to *begin* the diet.

My food plan works on a two-faced principle:

1. Nothing is specifically forbidden.
2. There is a list of sort-of-taboo foods that you as the wife or food preparer should be aware of but that your husband should never hear about. You can, of course, break the rules for special occasions. (I do!) As a general principle, you will no longer regularly buy, cook with, or use these products. And please avoid them totally for the first two weeks of the plan:
   • avocados
   • butter
   • canned vegetables or fruits ("lite" brands are okay)
   • candy
   • fatty pork products (bacon, breakfast sausage, etcetera)
   • ground meat (except for ground chicken, turkey, or veal)
   • half-and-half; heavy cream
   • hard liquor, except for light wine
   • hot dogs (even chicken dogs)
   • ice cream
   • ketchup
   • mayonnaise (use plain yogurt instead)
   • munchies (chips, pretzels, etcetera)
   • pasteurized cheeses and cheese spreads
   • pre-cooked meals (as in TV dinners), except for those discussed on pages 112–13, and if you can live without them, better yet
   • processed luncheon meats, even turkey
   • soft drinks (diet or otherwise)

- store-bought baked goods and desserts
- sugar-coated (or honey-coated) cereals
- sugary spreads and toppings ("lite" brands are okay in moderation)
- Vitamin D milk
- white bread

Trick or Treat: Grocery Shopping

That list may look upsetting, but if you analyze it carefully, there aren't any real surprises . . . except maybe ketchup. You didn't know about all the sugar in ketchup, did you? I don't care if you —or your husband—dip a few fries into the ketchup on a day out at a fast-food joint, but if you come from a family (or have a man bred by the Army) that hides the taste of food under ketchup, you have a problem. Mustard is okay; ketchup is not!

For the foods on the taboo list, please note the many substitutions. "Lite" products are usually preferred to "heavy"; plain yogurt works just as well as mayonnaise yet has fewer calories (100 calories per *tablespoon* of mayo; 140 calories for a full eight ounces of plain yogurt!). Sometimes synthetic "diet" products do the trick—like a whipped topping for a special-occasion dessert rather than whipped heavy cream and sugar. As you get to know the taboo list better, you'll get to know the list that follows even more intimately and learn to make creative substitutions—the fine art of "substitutionary locomotion." It's just juggling, so don't panic.

As you change your cooking and serving style

to accommodate this food plan, you'll find yourself changing your shopping habits as well. You may even be making more trips to the grocery store, or finding other markets, to round out your search for inventive, low-calorie foods.

Luckily for all of us, the grocery store is in a state of flux. More and more gourmet foods are being shipped to everyday markets all over the country. You no longer need to live in one of the five biggest cities or go to a fancy, overpriced market to find the new and exciting foods. But different markets do get different brands. As a result, I now use three supermarkets—all are in my neighborhood and are no more special than what you have in yours—since it takes three stops to fill out my shopping list with the different brands I sometimes need. If you have ethnic markets in another part of town, take some time on a weekend to investigate, especially any Oriental markets.

When you go to the supermarket, you should have an item-for-item shopping list to help you avoid overbuying and impulse purchases. If it's not on your list, try not to buy it. When you haven't time or energy for proper shopping, have some meals in the freezer you can fall back on. You may want to consider forming a meal co-op. Never run into the market and buy what's easiest just to throw something on the table. You'll end up starting a bad habit that can sabotage the entire food plan. You must do your shopping strategically; never shop when you are too tired to cope. Never take the responsibility for your husband's weight lightly . . . or you'll end up seeing him step on that scale not so lightly.

Next time in the market why don't you try a few of my favorite things:

- cilantro (Chinese parsley)
- Dijon-style mustard
- farmer cheese, ricotta cheese, skim milk cheeses
- fiber-heavy breads (whole wheat, seven grain, etcetera)
- fresh herbs
- lite products (including lite wine and beer)
- low-fat dairy products (like cottage cheese, etc.)
- low-fat milk (2% milk)
- plain (unflavored) yogurt—no fruit flavors, fancy flavors, or even vanilla
- popcorn (without butter and salt, of course)
- poultry (except duck or goose)
- safflower oil
- seafood
- seltzer (Canada Dry)
- vegetable cooking spray (instead of oil)
- raindrops on roses

How to Read a Label

Although labels are written in English, they usually make as much sense as a chemistry text. But there are a few basic rules that can help you know what you are buying. Remember the most important rule: The ingredients *must* (by law) be listed in the order of quantity, so the greater the amount of any ingredient, the closer it is to the beginning of the list. Here's the catch; there are many different products and byproducts that are basically the same thing—hence a product high in sugar may not be labeled sugar 57%, but instead could say sugar 22%, dextrose 19%, fructose 11%, corn syrup 3%, etcetera.

Other names for sugar include sucrose, dextrose, lactose, molasses, honey, corn syrup, fructose. Just because a label says *no sugar* doesn't mean that the product isn't fattening or that a sugar substitute wasn't used. Sometimes real sugar is better for you than the substitute. Be very wary of *no sugar* products. There is a relatively new product called *aspartame* (sold commercially as NutraSweet), which is an amino acid combo that provides sweet taste and few calories. However, it has not been on the market very long and no long-range testing has been done. While the notion of making a chocolate cream pie with hundreds of calories fewer per serving is enticing, it is currently impossible to know how much aspartame the body can safely ingest. My old-fashioned sense of things says to use this product in moderation and watch for updates on it in the media. Meanwhile, move your family's eating patterns away from sweets altogether.

Low-calorie and reduced-calorie do not mean the same thing; low-calorie means there are no more than forty calories per serving, and the package tells you the size of that serving. Reduced-calories means that there are one-third fewer calories than the regular product—lite brands are reduced-calorie products.

Low-sodium means that there is less salt in the product than before, but there is still salt in it. Many low-sodium products do not taste terrific—experiment brand by brand before you spend a lot of money. Preparing a low-salt or salt-free version of faux-gourmet food is not difficult. If you don't like low-sodium products, don't despair—you can still meet your dietary needs and have good food with other products.

Diet Products

Since the early 1950s, diet products have proliferated. They used to taste worse than the package they came in. Now many are quite sophisticated. The pressure to stay slim, and the competition from diet and lite foods, has made many manufacturers label the calorie count of their product, whether it is a diet product or not. Many products that you think have a high calorie count, do not. (I allow a dish of chocolate pudding made with low-fat milk . . . about 150 calories.) Or many fattening foods are not as fattening as you thought they were and can easily be worked into a 2,000-a-day calorie budget.

While I have sampled many diet products in my search for the perfect 500-calorie meal, my personal rule of thumb is to avoid products made with fake anything. Even though many diet foods taste great, I avoid them except for a few odd personal choices. (I love Weight Watchers ice cream sandwiches.)

When questioning a new product, read the label carefully, then test it for taste and performance. Just because a product has the word "diet" on it, or "low-sodium" or "low-cal," does not mean it tastes good or is healthy. The point of this food plan is that you serve great-tasting meals so your husband doesn't feel deprived. If you substitute inferior-tasting products, he will certainly catch on and rebel.

The Great Kitchen Lockout

Now that you've given grocery shopping a new meaning, it's time to reorganize your kitchen.

If you are able to put your entire family on this food plan, the kitchen reorganization will be easy: simply dump the old fattening foods and wave good-bye. Clean out the cabinets while you're at it (or bribe one of the kids to do it for you), then restock and restrict. The kitchen and its cabinets are now your private domain; hopefully you'll be able to keep everyone out—especially your man.

If you have teenage kids, particularly boys who are active in sports and who need a large number of calories, you'll have to divide up the territory and keep the snacks, goodies, and extras in a separate area. You must tell your children not to bring foods from this area to the table during regular meal times and not to snack in front of their dad. After school is the perfect time for your kids to snack, but remember to lead them to complex carbohydrates, rather than empty calories and sweet treats. (When in doubt—serve spaghetti!)

Barbi Benton, a local starlet, says she took weight off her husband by actually locking him out of the kitchen. She put padlocks on each of the cupboards. While I find this expensive, troublesome, and undecorative, it did work for Barbi. I prefer the modified lockout, which operates with words rather than hardware.

I told my husband we were beset by some kind of grain fly. This meant I had to (a) throw out everything we owned; (b) use a bug fogger and spray; (c) reline the cabinets; and (d) restock. I stretched out the time period from when I "discovered" the problem to the completion of the new improved cabinets to cover a full ten days, two weekends and a work week. During that period there was very little to eat in our house and absolutely no packaged goods could be bought.

Since I had already observed that my husband's biggest sin was bedtime snacking, eliminating snack foods was a big help. I also defrosted the freezer and got rid of the ice cream, frozen Snickers, Popsicles, and other treats.

For the first two weeks of the plan, the cupboard was bare. Sure, I got complaints from Mike and the peanut gallery. But I weathered the criticism, the grumblings, and the whining with careful persistence in my story—those damn grain flies! I was sympathetic to my boys; I was sorry it was taking me so long, but I was *terribly* busy with so many things, I was doing the best I could, etcetera, etcetera. And everyone survived. Except, of course, the grain flies.

You do not need an excuse to clean out your kitchen shelves, dump foods your family shouldn't be eating, or reorganize your system. I wanted to buy as much time as possible with the minimum of food in the house, then I gradually stocked up as I saw what weight loss methods were working on Mike. The ideal plan is to go the first two weeks with as few supplies as possible, so that even if your man is rebelling against the diminished intake, there is little he can do about it. Most snackers eat what is at hand. (Some will get in the car and drive for more food, *but not many.*) And since men are used to having their food provided for them with easy access, they are not all that likely to go out in the dead of night for ice cream and cookies. If he does go buy something, you probably won't be able to store it due to the problem with the grain flies and the pesticide, or it will melt when the freezer is defrosted. Without any elaborate explanations of what's going on, just keep tossing whatever new foods arrive. Yes, this is wasting money, but the cost of your husband's casket will be even steeper. And don't you forget it.

Say Good-Bye to Snack Time

For most men, a change in snack routines (that is, elimination) can achieve the loss of ten pounds. For the first two weeks, snacks should be banished totally. After that, you will have to punt. Snack times find their way into a day's schedule insidiously, so you have to look for them, check your husband's eating patterns, find out exactly where he's guilty, and then get to work. It pays to be paranoid about snack time—it is always sneaking up on you. The snack times that you can have no control over—the ones related to his work and business—you should not attempt to interfere with. Home snacks can successfully be wiped out for the first two weeks of the program and possibly forever. I like to think a snack is a treat for a special occasion. Convince your husband.

If less *is* more, you've got to start somewhere.

Priority Lists

As you become familiar with calorie counts, you will be able to make quick priority ratings. This means that within seconds your brain will tell you to reach for the chicken rather than the steak while you are surveying the market's meat bins. Or you'll come to know how to choose the lesser

84

of two fattening evils when deciding on a dessert
—a piece of pie is to be preferred to a dish of ice
cream. (No ice cream on the pie, either!)

Say you are preparing a tuna sandwich. Calorie
budgeting would teach you that it's a great idea
to use only one piece of bread, thereby saving 75
to 100 calories. Priority rating would tell you it's
better to use whole wheat bread than white; better to use low-fat yogurt instead of mayo.

For each type of food, there is usually a choice
—one choice may just be smarter than the next.
You may find it more rewarding to eat something
different from what you planned.

Note: Priority lists are for calorie budgeting,
not for making nutritional decisions. However, if
the food is high in fat, it has a star next to it. I
would rather go for higher calories and lower fat,
personally, but that choice is up to you. I have
included the higher-fat items so you can learn
about them and juggle them accordingly.

There are more complete calorie lists at the
back of this book. These priority lists are merely
to teach you the valuable lessons of "substitutionary locomotion." If just about any dessert will
do, substitute a less caloric one; if you want a
piece of fruit, grab a Bosc rather than a Bartlett
pear, and so forth.

MEATS	CALORIES
veal scallopini, 3 slices (approximately .29 pound total)	60
chicken, fried drumstick, 1	88
chickenburger, 6 ounces, 1	90
veal chop, 1	100
chicken, ½ small	120
beef frank,* 1	140

85

MEATS   CALORIES

sausage links,* 3	210
flank steak, broiled, 4–6 slices (4 ounces)	220
lean chuck,* chopped, 1 cup	240
Beef liver,* cooked in sherry, approximately 6 ounces	260
turkey, 3.5 ounces	260
beef stew, with veggies, 1 cup	280
duck,* 3 ounces	300
pork chop,* 1 (with bone, approx. 3 ounces)	305
roast leg of lamb, 2 slices (6 ounces approx.)	311
rib lamb chops, 2 (meat only, 2 ounces each chop)	360
baked ham,* 1 large slice	369
spare ribs* in barbecue sauce, 4–5 (½ pound)	432
corned beef,* 6 ounces	633
roast beef,* 1 serving (8 ounces)	1000
club steak,* 9.8 ounces	1262
T-bone steak,* 10.4 ounces	1395
porterhouse steak,* 10.6 ounces	1400

BREADS   CALORIES

†'s indicate lowest nutritional value.

sesame bread stick†, 1	38
whole wheat, 1 slice	60
honey wheat, 1 slice	60
cracked wheat, 1 slice	66
Jewish-style rye, 1 slice	75
white,† 1 slice	75
raisin with nuts, 1 slice	95
matzoh, 1 piece	110
English muffin, 1	130
English muffin, cinnamon raisin, 1	140
hamburger bun,† white, 1	160

VEGETABLES   CALORIES

celery, 1 stalk	7
Boston lettuce, chopped, 1 cup	8
radishes, 10 medium-sized	8

VEGETABLES	CALORIES
romaine lettuce, chopped, 1 cup	10
cucumber, sliced, 1 cup	15
green cabbage, raw, 1 cup	17
asparagus, steamed, 6 spears	20
mushrooms, 1 cup	20
carrot, 1 medium-sized	21
red cabbage, sliced, 1 cup	22
tomato, 1	25
cauliflower flowers, 1 cup	30
eggplant, 1 cup	40
spinach, 1 cup	40
broccoli, 1 cup	56
chayote squash, 1 medium-sized	56
artichoke, steamed	67
corn on the cob, 1 medium-sized	72
new potato, boiled in skin, 1	100
Idaho potato, baked, 1 medium-sized	140

FRUIT (FRESH)	CALORIES
Grape, 1 green seedless	3½
apricot	20
peach, 1 medium	45
nectarine, 1 medium	46
cantaloupe, 1 cup melon balls	50
strawberries, 1 cup hulled	55
red raspberries, 1 cup	70
star fruit (Carambola), 1 medium	75
pineapple, 1 cup cubes	80
blackberries, 1 cup	84
pear, Bosc	85
blueberries, 1 cup	90
apple, 1 with skin	90–120
banana	100
apricots, 12 dried	100
papaya, 1 medium	120
mango, 1 medium	150
pear, Bartlett	200
figs, dried, 4 ounces	300
raisins, 4 ounces	325
avocado, 1 medium California	350

A slice of cake or pie represents ⅛ of the whole.

chocolate brownie cookie	57
gingersnaps, 3	90
fudge (chocolate), 1 ounce	113
animal crackers, 10	120
Twinkie, 1	140
angel food cake, 1 slice	148
lemon custard, ½ cup	150
carrot cake, frozen brand (no topping), 1 slice	152
apple walnut cake, frozen brand, 1 slice	152
chocolate pudding, ½ cup	165
pumpkin pie (no topping), 1 slice	185
ice milk, 1 cup	200
chocolate swirl pound cake, 1 slice	215
apple pie, 1 slice	250
cheesecake, 1 slice	250
ice cream, 1 cup	250–350
fried cherry pie, packaged, 1	420

SPREADS, TOPPINGS, CONDIMENTS   CALORIES

mustard, Dijon-style, 1 tablespoon	15
sugar, 1 teaspoon	20
tomato sauce, 1 teaspoon	25
salad dressing (low-cal), 1 tablespoon	25
barbecue sauce, 1 tablespoon	25
honey, 1 teaspoon	25
peanut butter, 1 teaspoon	45
cream cheese, 1 tablespoon	52
jam, 1 tablespoon	55
salad dressing, 1 tablespoon	85
mayonnaise, 1 tablespoon	140
sour cream, ½ cup	165
béarnaise sauce,	175
butter, 1 ounce	230
margarine, 1 ounce	230
olive oil, 1 ounce	270
safflower oil, 1 ounce	270

Vitamin Supplements

Vitamins happen to be a highly controversial subject. I have an old-fashioned theory about them, learned in my old-fashioned childhood. My mother was a pharmacist's daughter—she believed in vitamins; my father is a doctor—he said if you ate a well-balanced meal, you eliminated the vitamins. (He didn't put it that politely, but I don't want to embarrass him now.) As a result of this medical opinion, and the very simple experiment of taking a few vitamins and noticing that my urine turned bright yellow, I have never been an advocate of vitamin pills.

Over the past ten to fifteen years, some doctors, nutritionists, and lay people have taken it upon themselves to prescribe vitamin-supplement therapy. Now doctors are seeing many medical conditions that are the result of overdoses of vitamin pills.

If you feed your family well-balanced meals from the basic food groups, no one should need vitamin pills. On a 2,000-calorie-a-day food plan, your man should not need vitamin pills. If you believe that a one-a-day multiple vitamin can't hurt, I don't want to take that security away from you. But if you—or your man—are taking megadoses of vitamin supplements, please consult a doctor.

5

MAN'S BEST FRIEND (A WOMAN, NATCH)

My New Best Friend

Whoever suggested that man's best friend was a dog? Probably a jealous mother-in-law. The woman who cares enough about her man to buy this book and use this food plan is the best friend a guy will *ever* have. And that includes Mum.

Many men consider themselves too busy making the world safe for democracy to worry about important things like what they put in their mouths or when they last exercised. (Notice what a good job they've done with the world situation *and* their waistlines.) Women, who aren't supposed to worry their pretty little heads with affairs of state, are often left to be their husband's best insurance policies. So it should come as no surprise when I suggest that *you* learn about the good and bad foods. Keep an ignorant husband away from the kitchen, away from food, even away from dirty dishes (he may lick the plates). Be his best friend.

Mike and I have evolved our own system.

When he is confronted with a food choice, whether in a restaurant or at home, he reels off a list of possibilities. I give him the priority rating in terms of calories, nutritional value, and my weekly food plan. For instance, I might say, "Why don't you have the liver, since I rarely make it, and you haven't had meat in several days?" I doubt that your man will take the time to learn what he should be eating, but he may become savvy enough to allow you to help him, once you are out of your Sneaky mode.

As you learn more about food, you will be able to do your grocery shopping, cooking, and entertaining with ease. I don't expect you to memorize the next section of the book, but a good bit of it will stick to your memory just as grocery prices do.

When I worked for *People* magazine, there was a saying that described the best qualities of a cover subject: "Young is better than old. . . . Pretty is better than ugly. . . . TV is better than movies. . . . Music is better than sports. . . . Anything is better than politics." With that litany in mind, you will soon be priority rating your meals like this: "Chicken is better than meat. . . . Steamed is better than boiled. . . . Fresh is better than frozen. . . . *Anything* is better than fried."

Meats

I am a meat and potatoes person, so I tell you this with sorrow: red meat is not particularly good for you. Hopefully, you already know this sorry fact, so it doesn't come as too great a shock. Meat is hard to digest; it's fatty; it's mostly unnecessary.

While a man may define his masculinity by how big a steak he can consume, he will live a lot longer if he concentrates on chicken and fish. As a rule of thumb, I allow red meat once a week. By red meat I mean beef, pork, and lamb, but not veal. (So you may have lamb and veal in the same week.)

Pork has about the same fat content and calories, but if I had to choose between a pork chop or a steak, I'd take the steak. You may want to vary a week's menu with a lean pork roast or perhaps a ham, but try to avoid ground pork and sausage totally—they have a very high fat content.

If your man insists on some bacon with his flapjacks on his birthday—great—happy birthday. But bacon is *just* for special occasions!

When it comes to beef, please eliminate chopped beef, no matter what grade. If it is a special occasion like a big family cookout or the chili cookoff, use the specially ground, lean beef (or ground turkey or veal)—often the market will keep the fat content to 2 percent. (That means 2 percent additional fat in the package; it does not include the natural fat in the meat itself.) Hamburgers are *not* a necessary part of the new improved food plan. There really is life after beef burgers. Try to eliminate them from your husband's menu. Or make him veal, turkey, or chicken burgers.

While lamb is a nice substitute for beef on occasion, do not switch to lambburgers (one of my husband's favorites), because they, too, have a high fat content. Leg of lamb, lamb chops, rack of lamb, or lamb kebabs are all fine . . . once a week

92

as your red meat quota. Lamb chops are a favorite in my family; they are great for this food plan because they are small. Limit consumption to two. A kebab is also a clever way to restrict the amount of meat served without your husband's noticing he's been shortchanged.

With beef as expensive as it is, your pocket-book will be relieved to cut down on red meat. Remember to choose lean meats (flank steak is the leanest beef) and to cut away fat. Choose meats that can be served by the slice rather than by the unit (unless small chops are available), so you can serve less and make it look appetizing. Men like to eat a whole steak, so save the steaks for special occasions.

Chicken and Fish

Chicken and fish are going to be the mainstays of your new life, unless you are going vegetarian. (If you are already vegetarian, it's unlikely you're overweight.) If you do not already eat a lot of chicken, congratulations, you are about to begin. There are so many different ways to cook chicken that I could eat it just about every night—which is something I will not be asking of you or your husband.

If chicken is not a favorite, try other kinds of poultry: turkey a la Thanksgiving, ground turkey, turkey breast, turkey chili, sliced turkey from the deli, smoked turkey (but not too often on smoked poultry), or rock cornish game hen. Duck is too fatty, so save that for special occasions (Chinese New Year is a wonderful time for a Peking duck); the same for goose (Christmas only, please).

93

Smoked foods are still being studied as a possible link to certain types of cancer, so limit them to once or twice a month. (You're not supposed to be smoking so why should the chicken be allowed?)

I used to like fish, but I can't remember when or why. I know that when I was pregnant, the smell nauseated me, and I have never quite recovered. As a result, I have not had a piece of fish in some five years. Your husband, on the other hand, may like fish—or grow to like it. If you've got a man who adores fish, he is probably already thin and planning to live to be one hundred. Just don't fry his little gilled friends. Although there is much controversy about the high iodine content in shellfish and whether or not they can be safely eaten in moderation, shellfish do add variety to any food plan. Do not, however, equate shellfish with fish. Fish is much healthier.

Never buy shellfish from that man who sells lobsters, clams, and shrimp from the back of his truck at cut-rate prices—you may get hepatitis. But by all means feed your family as many fruits of the sea as they will eat. And go out for sushi (yes, raw fish can transmit parasites, so go to a well-known and clean sushi bar). Shellfish and sushi are expensive, which will help keep you from, excuse the expression, going overboard on them.

Veggies

There are very few veggies that aren't good for you. (An avocado is a fruit.) The best way to eat a vegetable is raw; the next best way is steamed.

The least attractive method of eating your daily greens is via frozen or canned products. Canned goods are often packed with sugar, salt, and preservatives. If you must choose between them, pick frozen. Many packages announce that the vegetables were quick-frozen—this may insure that the produce is almost as fresh as what you buy in the produce department. Read the package. If you are stocking a cabin in the Yukon, buy lite or low-sodium canned goods.

If at all possible, grow your own vegetables; you'll gain the many nutrients that are usually lost in shipping. If you live in an area that does not get much fresh produce anyway, a garden would be a real victory.

I happen not to like vegetables very much; even cooking them for other people bores me. Luckily, I met Frieda Caplan who is the queen of the fruits and vegetables. Mrs. Caplan, a Los Angeles-based fruit and vegetable broker (Frieda's Finest), imports and distributes weird— make that unusual—fruits and vegetables to groceries, not just fancy gourmet shops in metropolitan cities, but A & P's, and so forth all over the country. Through Frieda, I began to experiment with fruits and vegetables I had never heard of or seen before. I discovered cactus leaves, fiddlehead ferns, *haricots vert*, yellow Finnish potatoes, *feijoas, cherimoyas, arugula, radicchio,* and many other exotics, all of which added excitement to the dinner table and the palate. All were healthy and low-calorie. Frieda is forever conscious of the waistline, often provides free recipes in her packages, and publishes a newsletter that will entertain and educate you. (You can get the newsletter for about fifteen dollars a year. Write for details to Frieda Caplan, Frieda's Finest, 732 Market Court, Los Angeles, CA 90021.)

Served raw or steamed, most vegetables have very few calories and little fat. If you drown them in butter, cheese, sauce, or mayonnaise, you will get fat. If your husband insists on having a little something over his veggies to mask their identity, make a salad dressing or mustard sauce (Dijon mustard and low-fat yogurt) or yogurt dip. Forget you ever learned how to pronounce the word *béarnaise;* do not put butter on the table. Try new salads, crazy combinations, and ethnic specialties to jazz up a meal. And remember, if you are attempting to fill out a plate or bulk up a meal—do it with veggies!

User-Friendly Fruits

Most people think fruits and vegetables are equally low-calorie—in other words, that they can eat all the fruit they want without gaining weight. *Wrong!* Fruits are fattening because they have a good bit of natural sugar. A piece of fruit is not as fattening as a brownie, but if you are trying to lose weight, it pays to know which fruits are user-friendly. (See priority rating page 87.)

Orange juice is very fattening; grapefruit juice is a better choice, with half the calories. Tomato juice has half the calories of grapefruit! Apple juice is almost as high as orange juice. Frozen juices traditionally have fewer vitamins and more calories than fresh: Six ounces of fresh-squeezed Valencia orange juice has 85 calories versus 120 calories for frozen Snow Crop. An orange has fewer calories than a glass of juice.

Fruits are good for your body and are a far better choice than junk food, packaged sweets, baked goods, etcetera. But don't think that fruit is a "free" food.

If you are bored with the same old fruits you've been eating since childhood, try ethnic markets and markets that do business with Frieda . . . but watch the calorie count. It's great to experiment with something new, but not if it has 300 calories per unit! The Priority List on page 87 will give you a good idea which fruits are worth spending money on. After a recent election, a prominent senator was asked how he kept his weight down while on the campaign trail. He confessed this fabulous secret: He ate lots of cantaloupe and only picked at the rest of the food served him throughout the day.

Dairy Products

Every balanced meal needs dairy products, but some of these are more fattening than others. Take cheese, for example. You might think that cheese makes a great snack, is terribly healthy, and is ideal for rounding out a dietetic meal. Well, the cheese stands alone, folks. Most cheeses are very high in calories and fat because of the milk from which they are made. Cheese is just another version of butter! The creamier the cheese, the more fattening it is. Watch the *triple crèmes!*

If you are a cheese lover, look for cheese made of skim milk. Some diet cheeses taste awful, but because manufacturers know that tremendous profits lie ahead for the person who creates a delicious dish with fewer calories, there are new products coming out all the time. Keep testing and asking around. Check out the new faux cheeses that are called "cheese spreads" or "cheese-style foods."

Cottage cheese is another story. Sure, if you eat too much of it you can grow to hate it on sight, but it *is* low in calories and high in nutritional value. Stay away from creamed cottage cheese—too much fat. Ricotta is also a good choice, as is farmer cheese.

Milk need not be eliminated from anyone's diet, but it should be low-fat (2%). Some people think drinking skim milk will guarantee them a place in the Dieters' Hall of Fame. I think skim milk is disgusting to look at and to drink (why does it always have a bluish tinge?). The difference between skim milk and low-fat milk in terms of fat content is three grams, yet the taste and appearance differences are tremendous. Here is the place to splurge. You're not supposed to be suffering on this food plan, so drink skim milk only if you happen to prefer it. (Pervert.) Also use low-fat milk in cooking, with cereal, and in coffee (rather than half-and-half or nondairy creamers). Avoid synthetic milk whenever possible. Powdered milk is exactly the same as regular milk, calorie-wise.

Eggs have become a confusing subject, since many contradictory opinions have been offered over the past ten years. Many of the anti-egg people are more against eggs for men than for women. (This has to do with estrogen and therefore bears no relevance to your husband's waistline.) I hover in the middle of the hen house: I don't think your man needs two eggs each and every day, but I am not against two eggs twice a week. Omelets are a good way of feeding a man a heap of healthy food in an attractive, one-dish meal.

The time to worry about cholesterol is during a man's early years—twenty to forty. If he has a high cholesterol level at that age, proper diet may, indeed, help save his life. As men age, a higher level does not constitute as great a risk, and by age sixty-five, is no longer a particular problem. The theory is that some bodies naturally rid themselves of excess cholesterol and some do not. If your man's body does not, you need to know as early as possible to prevent clogged arteries. If his body is running its own search-and-destroy mission, you needn't worry.

If your husband has high cholesterol, talk to your doctor and get several opinions from various experts. If he does have a problem, investigate egg substitutes. I am not crazy about their taste, but I would *grow* to love them if my husband's life depended on it. You may also consider this trick: in recipes that call for several eggs, eliminate one or two yolks from the total . . . the cholesterol is in the yolk, you know.

Don't fry your eggs or serve them over ham and under *béarnaise* or *hollandaise* sauce; do think up clever ways to make them exotic. I've seen eggs poached with asparagus or broccoli, or served with a dash of caviar. No man is going to complain about breakfast fare like that!

Dessert

There are men who can lose weight merely by cutting out all desserts. I think dessert makes any meal more of a celebration. Besides, as you try to please your husband with this new style of cooking and eating, you will find dessert goes a long way in convincing him he ate a whole meal.

You, as a woman, should stay away from dessert if you are trying to lose weight. On a man's 2,000-calorie-a-day meal plan, however, carefully thought out desserts are allowed. Your husband may not like the way I define dessert, but I do promise him a treat at the end of the meal. I prefer dessert after dinner—not lunch. Lunch can be a bigger meal anyway, and it's mostly beyond your control. Dessert after dinner is part of the budgeting of calories in my food plan, so don't even consider it a luxury.

Once your husband knows he is on a diet, he may volunteer to cut out dessert. Or he may prefer the dessert as a snack later in the evening. (He should *not* have both!) Mike and I were roaming around a mall one evening when Mike announced, "I'm having a chocolate-chocolate-chip and don't you say a word." (Ice cream is the most fattening of life's pleasures!) We went to the ice cream parlor where we bumped into some friends of ours. The wife had used my plan (she actually switched to vegetarianism), and her husband was now thirty pounds lighter. Mike declared it a special occasion, and we each had a dish of ice cream while they *shared* a dish. When you indulge, make sure it's not too often or too much.

In choosing dessert, fresh is best, so avoid buying packaged anything. Desserts should have fewer than 150 calories, which gives you a wide range but still eliminates the positively sinful. (Ice cream runs 250+ per scoop.) Dessert can be a piece of fruit, a sorbet, one or two cookies, a faux ice cream sandwich, or a creatively concocted small portion of something wonderful. I am not discussing a wedge of lemon meringue pie, a hot fudge sundae, or an entire Sara Lee boxed cake.

Dessert portions should always be small and pretty to look at. You can decorate them with paper parasols, doilies, frills, or store-bought geegaws. (Especially in the beginning weeks, the treat effect helps fool the tongue. Honest.) You are serving more promise than substance, so give it all you've got!

Here's a list of calorie counts on various desserts, so you can get a picture of how many choices are available:

D-Zerta chocolate pudding, one serving (½ cup)	20
Cherries, fresh, ½ lb. (that's a lot of cherries)	107
Alba chocolate milk shake, 1	113
Pepperidge Farm Bordeaux cookies, 3	117
Banana, large, 1	119
Apple, 1	123
Red raspberries, ½ lb., (serves four)	130
Baskin Robbins mango sherbet, 1 scoop	132
Sara Lee banana cake, 1 slice (if the whole cake had 8 slices)	132
Chips Ahoy chocolate chip cookies, 3	150
Hostess chocolate cupcake, 1	155

See pages 88 and 177 for more listings.

Junk Food

Junk food is basic to modern life. In modifying your husband's diet, you can still allow him some access to foods he loves, especially as a treat or when fast foods make *your* life easier. A few times a month, you should all be able to enjoy plastic serendipity.

Junk foods should be eaten outside the house. Never ask for a doggy bag; refrain from take-out.

I define junk food as anything riddled with empty calories, deep fried, or served from a red laminated tray. Fast food is invariably junk food —that includes the kind at restaurants and the kind frozen and reheated for consumption in front of a television.

When choosing junk food, look for the most nutritional products possible. Fried foods are high in fats; so are overprocessed foods, which include packaged sweets like those chocolate zingers my son adores. Pizza, on the other hand, is not a terrible choice—it's fresh bread, tomato sauce, cheese, and a topping. So the bread and cheese are a bit more fattening, big deal. If your man can stop at two pieces of pizza and a salad—he will survive. Or give him a fork and invite him to eat the topping off and leave the crust: You can hover around 500 to 600 calories using this method and still eat a plate-sized pizza. (Thin-crusted cheese pizza has 180 calories per slice; half a 10-inch cheese pizza has 450 calories.)

If you don't think junk foods are *really* damaging, take a look at this:

Super Brazier Burger	780
Large Fries	320
Double Whopper	850
Extra Crispy 3-piece Chicken Dinner	950
Big Mac	540

If you have a special occasion, or know that your man will be particularly active on a week-end, perhaps your calorie budget will allow him a junk food splurge. But looking briefly at the numbers, you can easily understand why a steady diet of these foods will make you "pudgy."

TIP: If you get a junk food craving, or if he gets one you don't know how to handle, try suggesting that you eat your carefully prepared meal and *then* go out for a junk food dessert. A glazed donut from Dunkin' Donuts is only 168 calories; the apple pie at Burger King is only 240 calories. If you serve a Lean Cuisine dinner of approximately 350 calories, you'll have the pleasures of not cooking, of going out on a date, and of eating half the calories.

Staying Alive

Mother was right: You are what you eat. But she had no way of knowing that in 1980 the National Cancer Institute would appoint a Committee on Diet, Nutrition and Cancer that would come up with preliminary advice and basic guidelines outlining the possibility of a link between cancer and certain foods! Various heart associations have also done research over greater periods of time, showing that certain foods may negatively affect your health.

It's not that one bite of these foods will kill you. Perhaps you know people who have eaten them steadily for fifty years and have lived to be one hundred. We all know of smokers who have lived to be ninety. Generally speaking, however, there are foods that could shorten your life if eaten habitually. And there are other foods that can help sustain your life. Here are some medically approved tips:

1. Reduce your consumption of both saturated and polyunsaturated fats. Only 30 percent of your total calories may be fat, not the current average of 40 percent.
2. Eat fresh fruits and vegetables, especially those rich in vitamins C and A and the cruciferous group (broccoli, cantaloupe, sweet potatoes, tomatoes, brussels sprouts, cabbage, carrots).
3. Take megadoses of nutritional supplements or vitamin pills only with a doctor's permission.
4. Avoid foods that have been salt-cured, salt-pickled, nitrate-cured, or wood-smoked, such as hot dogs, bacon, etcetera.
5. Reduce intake of salt, sugar, and sugar substitutes.
6. Drink alcoholic beverages in moderation only.
7. Do not smoke cigarettes or take drugs.
8. Reduce intake of coffee and caffeine-laden products.
9. Add fiber to your diet by eating fruits, vegetables, grain cereals, or unprocessed bran; eat baked goods made with whole-grain cereals.
10. Drink plenty of water (six to eight glasses per day).

Life-Shortening Foods

Fats

Polyunsaturated fats are from vegetables and are liquid at room temperature; this type of fat is thought to lower cholesterol in the bloodstream.

Monosaturated fats are also liquid at room temperature and vegetable in origin (examples include peanut or olive oil), but they don't seem to have any effect on cholesterol at all.

Saturated fats are animal in origin (except for coconut and palm oil) and are usually solid at room temperature. These are the fats that have been found to raise cholesterol content in blood.

Here are some foods that are particularly high in fats. You'll note that most have been discontinued from your regular shopping list already, because you are a conscientious wife and read the previous chapter.

High Fat: avocado, nuts, fried foods, meats, whole milk, cream cheese, processed cheese, hard cheeses, butter, margarine, cooking oils, cookies, cakes, pastries, pâté, mayonnaise, ice cream.

Medium Fat: garbanzo beans, soy beans, chicken, veal, kidney, liver, fish, peanut butter, canned soup.

Low Fat: fruits (except avocado), most vegetables, buttermilk, skim or low fat milk, cottage cheese, yogurt, breakfast cereals, pasta, rice, oatmeal, clear soups.

Life-Sustaining Foods

Don't panic, there's also a list of foods that are supposed to be especially good for you which you can derive from that list.

Cruciferous Vegetables

When the National Academy of Science's cancer report was made public in 1983, the word cruciferous jumped into the layman's vocabulary. A cruciferous plant is one that has a flower, like broccoli, cauliflower, brussels sprouts, and so forth. The medical research points to probable lower incidence of stomach, colon, and rectal cancer when cruciferous vegetables are a steady part of the diet. Supposedly, these veggies have certain chemical compounds, such as phenols, indoles, and isothiocyanates, that may have cancer-inhibiting effects. They also keep bowel movements regular, which helps clean out carcinogens that may have been consumed in other foods. They are high in vitamins and minerals. (If you are allergic or suffer from arthritis ask your doctor about the new supplemental pills.)

Fresh Fruits and Vegetables

There are more nutrients and more fiber in fruits and vegetables when they are fresh than when they are in any other form (such as canned or frozen).

To maximize the health benefits of fruits and vegetables, follow these tips:

1. Never soak them before cooking.
2. Eat them raw whenever possible.

3. Don't chop and store—nutrients are lost.
4. Avoid copper pans for cooking—they encourage oxidation and the loss of Vitamin C.
5. Keep cooking time as short as possible.
6. If you must cook, steam. Steaming retains more nutrients than other cooking methods.
7. Do not add salt or bicarbonate of soda to cooking water—this destroys vitamin C and B.
8. Eat vegetables as soon as you've cooked them; the longer they sit around, the more vitamins they lose.

If you have a history of allergies, consult your doctor and experiment with safe foods for you.

Fiber

Many experts believe that what is most wrong with the American diet is its lack of fiber. Fiber has been touted as the "lazy man's way to weight loss," because it's healthy and filling so that you "get full" faster without overeating. Fiber also passes through your body in a shorter period of time, so it doesn't stick to the ribs. It prevents constipation as well. The type of fiber you eat is important, however, so don't just down a bowl of shredded wheat and think you've done your duty. Get fiber from unprocessed bran, from beans, carrots, rolled oats, and fresh fruit. Buckwheat is a great source. Strawberries and raspberries are very high in fiber. You don't have to suffer to introduce a high-fiber ratio into your diet. Various experts suggest different amounts. I feel that four teaspoons a day of unprocessed fiber (preferably added to a diet that is a little higher in fiber than the average) will do the trick.

If you want more unprocessed fiber, check with your doctor first. Too much fiber—especially when gulped from a spoon—can make you sick.

Suzy's Top Ten Ways to Get Fiber Into His Life

1. Serve raspberries, strawberries, or blackberries as dessert.
2. Mix garbanzo beans into the salad.
3. Serve bran cereal at breakfast, then mix in a little unprocessed bran.
4. Serve corn on the cob (preferably fresh but frozen will do—on occasion).
5. Have dried apricots, figs, or dates for dessert.
6. Try buckwheat pancakes, crepes, or blini.
7. Eat baked potatoes with the skins.
8. Eat brown rice instead of white; forget instant rice no matter what color; try bulgur wheat or kasha.
9. Add raw broccoli to salad.
10. If you serve bread, make it multi-grain or whole wheat.

Even if you observe all ten of these tips, I still suggest that each member of the family over age twelve have four teaspoons of unprocessed bran a day, two in the morning and two at dinner or bedtime. I'm not talking about bran cereal, mind you, but unprocessed bran that can be bought for about ninety cents a box at a grocery or health food store. Bedtime bran can be enjoyed with a cup of herb tea and will be a respite from the troubles of the day. (I call this Leonard's Bedtime Treat, in honor of the friend who taught it to me. See the Water section that follows for methodology.) You can also mix bran with bouillon or instant soup, and serve about twenty minutes before a meal—this will not only add fiber to the body but will fill up your hungry man so he consumes less at the dinner table!

Water

We all know we're supposed to drink a lot of water because we learned it in fifth-grade science. Yet we never do. (If you drink eight glasses of water a day, go to the head of the class and skip this part.) Most people think drinking several diet sodas a day is equal to drinking plain old water—and a lot more exciting. Yes, it's more exciting, but that's the end of the story. Diet drinks may have few calories, but they are filled with chemicals and, sometimes, caffeine. Water may have some chemicals in it, but they're not as bad as those in diet drinks! (If your tap water is unhealthful for drinking, use filtered or bottled water.)

Water is good for you because it has no calories, aids in digestion and elimination, keeps your body temperature stable, and keeps your insides at peace with each other. Drinking water is also good for your skin and hair. You don't have to drink fancy bottled waters or spend a lot of money to make water more palatable. A good water filter on your kitchen tap should provide you with healthy water, or you can buy any of the plain or sparkling waters that are now stocked in grocery stores, or you can specifically look for no-sodium water, which is what I serve at home. (We like Canada Dry's Seltzer.)

We serve a combination of sparkling and plain water—the sparkling takes the place of a soft

drink and makes dinner more special. I sometimes buy A Santé, a flavored sparkling water
(lime, mint, or orange), or add a dash of flavored
oil or essence to a bottle of seltzer. (See the spice
department of your market.)

To get the amount of water you need to be
drinking, you probably have to force yourself and
your family to drink up. Our water schedule
looks like this:

Morning: two teaspoons of bran from a spoon before breakfast taken with eight ounces of tap
water. (It's not bad at all . . . sort of nutty and
chewy.) Another eight ounces of tap water with
breakfast.

Lunch: two glasses of water (eight ounces each).

Dinner: eight ounces seltzer or sparkling water.

Evening: another two teaspoons of unprocessed
bran washed down with eight ounces water or
sparkling water, or with a six- to eight-ounce
cup of warm water with lemon or with a six- to
eight-ounce cup of herb tea (see Leonard's
Bedtime Treat below).

Okay, so that's only six glasses of water. Get to
six, and then we'll discuss it further.

Here's Leonard's Bedtime Treat. Make up a
beautiful bedtime tray for your spouse: Place a
rose in a vase if possible, use a nice napkin and
a pretty tea cup. Serve a cup of herb tea (Leonard
says Sleepytime is the only brand to serve) and
two teaspoons of bran. No, you do not mix the

bran into the tea—the tea is to wash down the bran. This will help meet your water needs, your bran needs, and will serve as a blissful reminder that you care.

Special Foods

Here are some favorites I lean on heavily to keep Mike from leaning too heavily.

Flank Steak. If you're looking for meat, this is the leanest, least fattening choice. A pound of "choice" flank steak has very little fat and divides into servings of about 150 calories each.

Spinach. It must have been Olive Oyl who turned her man onto this diet food. Spinach is packed with vitamins and minerals; raw, it has only 26 calories per half-cup serving. You can eat it raw or steamed.

Cantaloupe. It's gorgeous to look at, refreshing when cold, and nice as part of a meal, as dessert, or as an hors d'oeuvre. Don't forget to use half a cantaloupe as the serving dish for a salad.

Pasta. Pasta itself isn't fattening. It's what you put on top of it that sends you to the tailor to let out your seams. I find pasta a great "sick" food or "blue" food—it seems to have healing properties second only to mother's chicken soup. There are lite pastas, but a five-ounce serving of spaghetti has only 210 calories. Whole wheat or vegetable pastas weigh in at about 200. Top with fresh zucchini and garlic, and you have a great, low-cal dinner. There are also lite spaghetti sauces with about 50 calories per serving. That's up to you.

Eggplant. Don't laugh but there's research (from the University of Graz in Austria) that eggplant, when served with fatty foods, helps absorb the cholesterol and carry it out of the digestive system. Just don't fry your eggplant!

Low-Calorie Shortcuts to Remember

• *Lite Is Often a Delite.* I had always considered diet foods to be inferior tasting and too expensive for serious consideration. In the last few years, however, they have been transformed and we have enjoyed the "lite" revolution. There is now a lite version of just about everything, so check for it before you use its "heavy" counterpart.

• *It's the Real Thing.* Sometimes the real product is not as fattening as you think it is. Try my little chocolate pudding experiment. Compare the information on the boxes of all the types of chocolate pudding—diet, fake, and old-fashioned — and you may find that regular, old chocolate pudding when made with low-fat milk yields a dessert portion that has fewer than 150 calories, which is well within your husband's dessert budget. Can you lose weight while eating chocolate pudding? Absolutely!

• *Frozen Low-Cal Dinners.* There are several newly introduced frozen dinners (Weight Watchers has a complete line, as does Stouffer's Lean Cuisine) that are low in calories and look appealing. I personally don't like many of these foods and serve them only when absolutely necessary, but you may have different taste buds. Check the labels; make sure they are low in salt. You certainly can't knock the convenience, the prices, and the calorie counts:

Weight Watchers Pizza ($1.69)	370 calories per serving
Lean Cuisine's Oriental Beef ($2.30)	280 calories per serving
Mrs. Paul's Light and Natural Fillet of Fish ($3.00)	290 calories per serving

Some Cautionary Advice

• *Artificial Sweeteners.* I am basically opposed to sugar substitutes because they are chemicals or amino acid compounds and, twenty years from now, your nose might fall off. But they can reduce the calorie content of a dessert by two-thirds, which is impressive. For special occasion desserts, I see nothing wrong with their use. (You cannot heat aspartame (NutraSweet), so its use is self-limiting.)

Products that have saccharin in them are now required by law to state that they could be hazardous to your health. It's much more sensible to cut back on sweets totally, or to eat natural sweets and forget sugar substitutes.

• *Egg Substitutes.* I do not use egg substitutes, but that doesn't mean you shouldn't. Your husband can get a cholesterol test during his next medical checkup. If his count is elevated, egg substitutes are probably a good idea. I have experimented with them to very mixed results.

• *Soft Drinks.* Just because a soda has the word *diet* on it does not mean that it's good for you. None of the popular drinks are *good* for you. Therefore choose the ones that are least offensive and cut down the frequency with which they are consumed in your family. One soda a day is a banquet. Serve caffeine-free and sugar-free versions of your favorite brands. Don't try to fill up on diet sodas. They add chemicals you don't need. But don't switch to fruit juices just because they are more healthful. They are very fattening, especially in quantity. Drink water! Or herb tea or iced tea, if you must. (No additional coffee, please.) Try a juice spritzer—half juice, half low-cal bubbly.

Priorities, Please

Eating and buying the right foods is largely a measure of education and care. Study the priority lists; do some experimenting; read labels carefully while shopping. You will soon conquer the main difficulty people face with a weight-loss program—its newness.

6

MEAL TIME

Substitutionary Locomotion

To show you precisely how less can be more, I will now teach you the art of substitutionary locomotion—swapping low-calorie, *faux gourmet* meals for high-calorie, old-fashioned meals. There is little difference in the bulk of the meals, so no one feels deprived, no one goes hungry.

Okay, here we go, your basic, old-fashioned, all-American lunch, for child or adult:

One peanut-butter-and-jelly sandwich made with two pieces of raisin-nut bread, three tablespoons of peanut butter and three tablespoons of grape jelly. You can't eat peanut butter and jelly without a glass of milk, can you? Add one eight-ounce glass of whole milk and, for dessert, two chocolate chip cookies. Total calorie intake (more or less): 750 calories! And most men would eat two sandwiches . . . total calories 1,250. That's a bit more than your basic 500-calorie budget, and it isn't even an exciting lunch.

Now then, hocus pocus, substitutionary locomotion. Try any of these *faux gourmet* lunches instead:

Six ounces of chicken and basil pasta salad, a glass of seltzer and one scoop of apple sorbet . . . 440 calories.

Eight ounces Suzy's Chopped Salad with home-made dressing (see recipe, p. 186); chocolate pudding; coffee or tea . . . 575 calories.

Two English muffin halves, each spread with two ounces of farmer cheese and two ounces of lean, smoked turkey breast; seltzer; Bosc pear . . . 515 calories.

The possibilities are endless. You just need to take the time to do the calorie budgeting and the grocery shopping—and use your imagination. The results are worth it: Meals are less boring *and* your man loses weight! I dare him to notice you've been playing with his lifeline.

Faux Gourmet Translated

My French and my cooking are on a par, which is far from sublime. I can cook a pleasant enough meal and read a French dinner menu, but that's about it. However, I do know the word for fake is *faux*—I learned it from my jeweler!—and I think it perfectly sums up the not-quite-gourmet fare I invented for my husband and our new low-calorie life-style.

As long as your meals are within the proper calorie budget, you can serve any style you want. You may not need the recipe section in this book or any of the numerous low-cal products and cookbooks now flooding the markets. Fine. But if you're looking to transform simple cooking to make it seem a little more special to the man who is about to take off twenty pounds, stick with me . . . and faux gourmet.

Excuse me, Julia Child, you go right on doing your own thing and *bon Noël* to you (I think that's Merry Christmas, I don't know the word for good luck). If *nouvelle* cuisine is your style, my best wishes and *bonne chance*. (There, I remembered it!); if *cuisine minceur* is your cup of *thé*, I am more than impressed with your oo-la-la. For the rest of us working moms, faux gourmet guarantees a healthy, low-calorie, tasty, and appealing meal on which our men can lose weight. You can't ask for anything more, can you?

Breakfast at Home

Ever since "Father Knows Best," "Leave It to Beaver," and "Lassie," we have known how to eat breakfast: Everyone sits at the table (in the sunlit dinette, of course) and eats orange juice, coffee, pancakes, bacon, and probably home-baked biscuits. Only in Lucy's family was the fare slightly different, because Lucy always burned the toast. It was at the breakfast table that Mr. Blandings (Cary Grant) found the slogan that saved his career ("If you ain't eatin' 'Wham,' you ain't eatin' ham."); it was at the breakfast table that we all learned how life was *supposed* to be lived.

We all sat down to similar breakfasts, cooked by Mom, who was, after all, a professional homemaker like Lucy and Harriet and Donna Reed. Those were the good old days.

Now that Mom's gone to work, and everyone's worried about the many calories in maple syrup (though lite maple syrup is now available, too), few families sit down to eat (a) together; (b) the same thing; (c) breakfast. In fact, only 15 percent of Americans even sit down to breakfast, period. The rest either skip it or eat on the go.

While you may survive without eating breakfast, I do not recommend it. If you are trying to take weight off your husband, he'll be a lot better off if he eats breakfast—and eats it under your tutelage. He should eat the heaviest meal of the day in the morning. As my mother-in-law once said, "Eat breakfast like a king, lunch like a prince, and dinner like a pauper." By eating progressively smaller meals during the day you are able to work off as many calories as possible before bedtime. This certainly beats the opposite system of skipping breakfast, eating a helter-skelter lunch, and having a gigantic dinner only hours before you go to sleep—with no chance of burning off that heavy meal.

On my food plan, everyone eats breakfast. It can be cereal (hot or cold), egg products, or a fruit protein drink. I'd save bready foods and batter dishes for special occasions or weekends. Never eat leftovers for breakfast.

Start each breakfast with those two tablespoons of unprocessed bran flakes, washed down with an eight-ounce glass of water. You may want to serve the bran and water while your man is shaving and performing his morning toilette, because the bran will expand and fill him up so that twenty minutes later, when he's ready for breakfast, he'll be rather full. Bran does not taste bad, honest.

You can include with his breakfast either a small (four- to six-ounce) glass of juice or a piece of fruit. Orange, grape, prune, and pineapple juice should not be served on a regular basis, but grapefruit (Seneca has only 55 calories per six ounces) or tomato juice are excellent choices. For fruit, an orange, banana, or apple is just fine, or a cup of raspberries, blackberries, or blueberries. Do not have *both* juice and fresh fruit. Do not substitute canned or frozen fruit if you can help it. See the priority listing for fruit on page 87 to get an idea of which fruits are least fattening; there is a very wide spread of calorie possibilities. (Never put sugar, cream, honey, or even milk on your fruit.)

If you choose a cold cereal, pick brands that are without sugar, NutraSweet, or honey and that are high in fiber. Skip the brands with raisins or dates. My husband mixes together his own concoction of Cracklin' Oat Bran, Grape Nuts (not Grape Nut Flakes), and Bran Buds. (He added Quaker 100% Natural Cereal with raisins only after he lost the weight.) Some health buffs mix their cereal with juice instead of milk. If this idea does anything for you, give it a try. It makes my stomach churn just to think about it. Remember, don't use orange juice because it's too fattening.

If you eat hot cereal, do not flavor it with an inordinate amount of salt, butter, margarine, sugar, honey, or milk. Every ounce of butter takes 100 calories from your budget. That's mighty expensive!

Make sure you use low-fat milk on your cereal.

Skip bread or toast, unless your meal is a sandwich.

If you are serving eggs, I allow two eggs unless I am serving a breakfast sandwich, then I go to one egg.

Eggs should never be fried. Basted, poached, boiled, or scrambled (with water, not milk) are the best choices. Use a Teflon or no-stick pan. Do not cook with butter or margarine; you can use a vegetable cooking spray called PAM, instead.

If your husband can go without his morning coffee, great. Otherwise serve him one cup only. If he is one of those people who seems drugged in the morning and claims to need several cups just to "wake up," he may require some other stimulus besides coffee (like exercise). There are people who bound out of bed in the morning and people who need to be dragged out, but most people get it together because they have to and can make do with a single cup.

I'm not pushing decaf coffee over caffeinated because the chemicals used in the decaffeination process are known to be harmful to laboratory animals. And, while I'm not one to fall into panic over the death of a few rats, if you—and your husband—can get along without coffee, why drink it at all?

If you make breakfast a sit-down, calm-down tradition, everyone in the family will have the benefit of a nice meal and a sensible way of digesting it. You may have to get up a half-hour earlier to pull this off, but you'll find it worthwhile. Try going to bed a half-hour earlier—with your skinny husband.

Weekend Breakfast

We used to love to start weekends off with the special treat of eating breakfast out. It turned out to be fattening and expensive, so we cut back in favor of special home-cooked weekend breakfasts.

On Sundays we ordered the *New York Times* to be delivered to our house. (This may not be a treat for you, but it is to us.) I cook a special meal, or Mike treks to the deli for bagels, cream cheese, and lox. This makes Sunday special, doesn't cost as much as a breakfast out, and makes Mike feel happily decadent—he can't believe that one-and-a-half onion and poppy seed bagels, with three ounces of whipped cream cheese and two small pieces of lox, are allowed on his calorie budget. (Okay, it's a little over 500 calories, but not much over, and since it's the first thing in the day, it'll get worked off later!)

It may also be helpful to you to invite people over for Sunday breakfast and prepare just barely enough food. If your husband is forced to eat a lighter than usual meal, he'll think it's because you were running out of food. This plan might work especially well for the first two weekends of the food plan when he doesn't know exactly what's going on.

Whatever your gimmick, it's nice to make your weekend breakfasts a little more special than your weekday breakfasts. It's also a chance to let your man eat some of the foods he thinks he has been missing. And if he happens to eat a few pieces of bacon, it won't kill him. (Bacon is the preferred choice to sausage links any day—sausage is twice as fattening.)

Breakfast Out: Business or Social

For some executives, breakfast in a restaurant is a way of doing business. They get up, leave the house, have a nice meal prepared for them, and don't have to pay for it. At the same time, they get some business accomplished.

For the man who eats breakfast out regularly, there is little he can do that will hurt him if he remembers to avoid

- fried foods (including eggs and potatoes)
- pork products (bacon, sausage, Canadian bacon, ham)
- breads—especially with butter and jam
- orange juice

He can eat

- eggs or omelets (not every day, though)
- one piece of French toast with any topping— he should stop after one piece
- a serving of fresh fruit or a glass of juice (not both and avoid orange juice)
- half an order of pancakes—he can leave the rest
- yogurt and fresh fruit
- cereal (hot or cold) but with low-fat milk, not heavy cream or half-and-half
- toast with cottage cheese and fresh tomatoes in an open-face sandwich
- one cup of coffee
- at least one glass of water

Lunch for the Average Businessman

The average white-collar businessman eats lunch at a restaurant near his office and rarely eats alone —he may have a business meeting or may eat with friends or colleagues. The last thing he ever wants to do is draw attention to his plate, his waistline, or the fact that he is attempting to lose weight. He just wants to be one of the guys.

Luckily, it's fashionable to eat healthy these days, so no one thinks twice if you order

- fish
- a luncheon salad
- sparkling water or wine, rather than hard liquor
- tomatoes, instead of potatoes
- cottage cheese, instead of whatever
- no dessert

A man who is beginning to be sophisticated about his food priorities can order a healthy and low-calorie meal without anyone noticing how careful he's been. He can even order dessert, have a few bites and put it aside as "too rich," etcetera. It's the uneducated man who gets into trouble. He's the one who is either eating in a hurry and depends on fast foods; who wants to take advantage of the fact that the business lunch is "free" and his wife certainly doesn't cook like that; who considers his lunch a reward for his hard day at work and doesn't want reality to muddle his delight; who wants to indulge and will feel deprived if he doesn't stuff himself.

How do you handle this man? Very, very carefully. In your observation period, you can get an inkling of his lunch attitudes and aptitudes. Meet him for lunch a few times; ask him questions about his lunches out. Husbands who go to fancy restaurants for lunch *expect* their wives to have voyeuristic thoughts about the meal, the restaurant, the diners, the prices, and so forth. You can ask a lot of questions (no, he won't remember what color the tablecloths were) and get a good bit of information merely by playing dumb. Once you know his lunch patterns, you can have a better idea of what can and can't be done.

Warning: Lunch is always going to be tricky, so it's a matter of what *can* be done. I don't expect you to be able to do much.

Ideally, you can insert yourself into his lunchtime at least on a part-time basis—get him to come home for lunch, meet you for a lunch date, or let you deliver his lunch to him. Perhaps he can be gently programmed by his secretary, so that some semblance of control is achieved. My husband and I work together, and while we don't eat together every day, I did see him more than usual for the first two weeks of the food plan— and it helped.

If you are using the Sneaky Approach, you may have to get some outside help. Either call the maitre d' at his usual hangouts, or get his secretary to steer him to restaurants where you know he'll get the kind of attention he needs. It pays to visit these restaurants yourself, tip the maitre d', and make very, very friendly to get the kind of help you need. Possibly the maitre d' will offer your husband some specials of the day that might not be on the menu, or suggest fish that is prepared simply, a special salad, or something else that can save several hundred calories.

If a business meeting is taking place, perhaps his secretary can pre-select a meal and order it ahead of time. This saves the men time and provides you with the opportunity to guide your husband away from heavier foods. (And if his secretary works on your team and helps with those luncheon arrangements, don't forget, when it's over, that big thank you or small gift.)

124

If it's totally impossible for you to get involved with his lunch in any way whatsoever, don't make yourself nuts. You'll still be able to take some weight off him.

Lunch from a Truck

For the average blue-collar worker, and for those in a hurry, lunch is invariably served from a truck. Some trucks actually have cooking facilities so they can grill a burger for you; many do not. Either way, his choices are limited and need to be made carefully. Since you, his guardian angel, aren't there to peer over his shoulder and guide him through these difficult decisions, you should do one of two things:

1. Let him eat whatever he wants.
2. Convert him to a brown bagger (good choice, woman!)

There is no peer pressure against brown baggers in this group, so you should have an easy convert. Even a combination of three days of brown-bagging with two days of trucking is better than all-week trucking.

Now here's a possibility that takes a little time and imagination, but could work out well for your man: Find a new supplier. Don't put the truck people out of business, that would be tacky, but get out your Yellow Pages and put your ear to the grapevine to find the names and numbers of the basket ladies. Basket ladies (not bag ladies) are very popular in Los Angeles. They go from office to office carrying cute picnic baskets loaded down with salads, sandwiches, and snacks that are usually health-food oriented. The prices are comparable to the truck food, but the quality is usually better. Just avoiding bread and mayonnaise will trim some 300 calories from your husband's lunch.

If your man is really serious about losing weight and is helping you with the effort, you may want to check out the lunch truck with him and help him find a priority rating. Or get him to bring his lunch.

Brown Baggers

If your husband takes lunch to work, you are both lucky. You will have no trouble controlling what he eats. (Unlike children, adults rarely swap lunch treats with their friends.) Make the lunch as attractive as possible, by including love notes or small diversions in his lunch box occasionally (a paperback book, a snapshot of the kids, a rubber spider, etcetera), using pretty napkins—making the meal as festive as possible, so instead of being a bore, it's fun and gives a psychological energy boost.

If your husband is partial to junk food, you can include teensy tiny samples—watch the size of the portion and the calorie content. There is a company that makes packs of potato chips that look very satisfying from the outside but open up to reveal only about four whole and two fragmented chips. Seriously, there is nothing there. If having something like a bag of chips in his lunch bag makes him feel better, these are the ones to buy! Careful calorie budgeting will allow you to feed him a good-sized meal and still titillate him with the junk food he loves.

Lunch can include a variety of elements and should total anywhere from 500 to 700 calories. You can do an awful lot with that as long as you don't serve pecan pie with whipped topping.

Here are some good things to put in a lunch box:

- thermos with soup (try a bran soup—healthy and filling)
- frozen can of juice that defrosts by lunch time but acts as a refrigerator
- pita bread sandwich
- kebabs of fruits or veggies
- mini salad bar
- ingredients for an open sandwich
- pasta salad
- low-cal deli foods
- sushi (if it is kept carefully refrigerated)
- lettuce rolls

Lunch Warning

You can lead your man to new trousers, but you can't make him skinny. In short, there is only so much you can do with this plan. If your man cheats on you at lunch, there really isn't anything you can do about it. Lunch will always be your weakest moment. Accept it and get on with the cooking. Because lunch is in the middle of the day, there is a chance that whatever sins he has consumed can be worked off. If you see that he is eating more than he should (or drinking more than he should) at lunch, if you see that even after an initial weight loss he cannot discipline his fork and mouth at lunch time, you may want to get him involved in an afternoon exercise program.

Admittedly, lunch is shaky ground. Go slowly; do a lot of watching and not much talking. As you implement the other changes in this book, see how he shapes up (or down, to be more precise), and adjust your expectations accordingly. Be clever about his lunches, but don't make yourself crazy.

Weekend Lunches

Weekend lunches are a drag. You're either forced to (1) use up leftovers that you feel morally committed to finishing; (2) eat fast foods that you know are fattening and non-nutritional but are easy; or (3) go in the kitchen and concoct something meaningful when all you want to do is escape from it all. As far as I am concerned, especially considering the intricacies and pressures of this food plan, there is no reason to cook lunch on the weekends.

1. Hopefully you will not be stuck with leftovers because you are no longer serving family style and have cut down the amount of food being served.

2. If your kids want fast foods, fine, let them— if that's part of your regular routine or life-style. If you can separate the kids' meals from yours conveniently, do so. If not, one fast-food meal isn't going to kill you or blow the whole diet. Weekends are the time for fast foods.

3. I prefer what I call European lunches: I buy a roasted chicken from the market or sliced turkey breast, an assortment of cheeses (choose

carefully because cheese *is* very fattening), fruits and vegetables, maybe a great bread (like onion dill whole wheat, something with a lot of flavor that's also good for you), and put it all on the table. **Warning:** Yes, this is family style, or buffet style to be precise, but you're going to put out just enough food to go around—barely—and you'll say something like, "I don't know if I bought enough, so go light." Round out with perhaps a dish of cottage cheese, some plain yogurt, and some Dijon mustard. It's help-yourself time. If I'm feeling very creative and loving about the food preparation, I may put the food in serving dishes or even incorporate much of it into a *salad*. But don't be surprised to come to my house and see the packages on the table. We all sit down and eat together, but it is not fancy!

Dinner at Home

According to the American Dream, every man is entitled to a Nice Dinner at Home. In post-war America, it was common for wives to stay home and prepare for this big event. Many women have since rebelled against this sometimes tedious task, often because they find it just too difficult to work all day and come home and prepare a special meal. They are forced to rely on fast foods, takeout places, frozen meals, and instant help.

To help your husband lose weight, you are going to have to plan meals carefully, dedicating about half an hour to their preparation. I know that hurts, but at least I'm honest. (Besides, when you think about it, *most* meals end up costing half an hour of your time.) I myself went through stages that seemed to last five days—some weeks I had tremendous enthusiasm and energy for the food plan; others I hated it and couldn't stand the time and calculation it required. On my hate weeks my husband didn't lose (he didn't gain either), but I got my spirit back in time to tackle the next week.

I've now been doing all this for so long that I can plan certain meals and table settings while my brain is on automatic pilot. You can't be creative every night of the week! After you get the hang of the food plan and the *faux gourmet* method, you too will find it can be done in your sleep.

Just remember, dinner at home is actually a two-part program:

1. The meal is low-calorie—a total of 500 to 600 calories.
2. Its presentation is dramatic, or special, or even elegant.

I don't mean that you should serve dinner on a flaming sword or do the hula when you bring out the casserole—but you will be putting as much effort into table setting and food presentation as you put into the actual cooking.

If you don't do the special effects, your husband might look down at the reduced amount of food and ask, "What's for dinner?" He may do this anyway, but it doesn't hurt to divert his attention.

If your husband does ask, "What the hell is going on?" you can tell him any number of truths or half-truths (or lies):

- You're taking a cooking class and are doing your homework.
- You saw the dish in a magazine and wanted to try it.
- You got bored with your life-style and wanted some cheap thrills.
- Your fantasy is to run a restaurant, and you're trying the art of presentation out on him.
- You think it's romantic; what's wrong with him?

I went for the I'd-like-to-run-a-restaurant routine, combined with our-life-is-so-boring. He fell for it. And now our life isn't quite so boring because he's slimmer and divine-looking.

To jazz up the dinner table, check "women's" magazines and home-furnishing magazines, browse through the library's books on entertaining, or try a few of my tricks:

- Serve dinner on a salad plate; place the salad plate on top of the dinner plate to fill up the space and make less look like more.
- Use parsley or other fillers as decoration.
- Put a little mound of lettuce with a slice of pineapple and a slice of melon and a slice of orange on the dinner plate to take up the room left by the lack of food.
- Buy cheap dishes at the swap meet or a garage sale to vary the table settings.
- Use paper and plastic party goods to get variety and excitement on the table, then toss (or rinse for future use). Combine paper and fabric as well.
- Use the silver, the china, the tablecloths you save for "good company" and therefore never use.

131

I've always found that flowers and centerpieces get in the way of the conversation, but if your table is big enough or looks empty without a lot of serving dishes, you might want to add this to the list. We eat at a smallish table in the kitchen, but if you have a big dining table, you may need to fill it with distractors. See what you can find at a discount party goods store, or pick flowers from your garden and place in individual-size vases at each place. Get creative with the use of placemats, tablecloths, and napkins—the joy you bring to the table will make the meal a more festive occasion. Don't forget candles—they're romantic and in the dim light he won't be able to *see* how little is on his plate.

While you're being creative, remember the McDonald's Rule: Hot colors make people hungry. The opposite is also true: Cool colors (or pastels) make people less hungry. So go for pale, restful, soothing color combinations; avoid reds, oranges, chrome yellows, and bright pinks. Dinner should feel like a summer breeze, not a sirocco.

If dinner is made into a special occasion, it is emotionally and physically more satisfying. I try to prolong dinner as long as possible, even excusing our son after the main meal is finished so we can linger over dessert. I don't believe in the eat-and-run theory, except during the World Series. The slower the meal, the more fulfilling.

I will occasionally serve dinner on a tray for Monday night football, but eating in front of the television set is a habit that should *not* be encouraged. (I've noticed on football nights that my husband will be very satisfied with a one-dish meal he can eat in a bowl. This is the perfect time to serve him yogurt or cottage cheese with chopped vegetables.) As a basic rule, though, TV meals are forbidden. (See Bad Habits, page 59.)

Quickie Dinner at Home

We all have our days, even weeks, when we just can't invest one ounce of extra energy in anything more than putting one foot in front of the next. Creating beautiful dinners is just too much to consider. I know all about it; I've been there too.

When you get into these ruts, as all of us do, you have several ways out:

1. Calorie-budgeted dinners you made and froze
2. Frozen low-cal dinners a la Lean Cuisine
3. Dinner out

Let's take them one at a time:

1. *Calorie-budgeted dinners.* Every now and then I experience an incredible energy high. I only get about four or five of these lightning strikes a year, and they normally last only a day or two. But when I have them, look out, world.

The next time *you* have one, why don't you prepare a series of calorie-budgeted meals you can wrap and freeze, ready to be defrosted and served at a second's (if you have a microwave) or an hour's notice? Even if you're not on an energy run, you can double your ingredients one night, serve half the food for dinner, then freeze the other half for another night. Buy plastic or foil dinner trays—just like the ones they had when we were kids and TV dinners were first invented

—and use heavy-duty aluminum foil for a tight wrap. Make a tray for each family member so you won't even have to worry about serving plates or dirty dishes later. Just defrost and warm in the oven.

2. *Frozen Dinners*. I keep several Lean Cuisine dinners in the freezer for those emergency times when I just can't *bear* the thought of even entering the kitchen. With the calorie count as low as 350 (check the box for the specific count), you may even be able to throw in a nice dessert—store-bought or frozen, of course—that will make everyone happy. Even if these meals aren't as nutritionally sound as I'd like them to be, they certainly won't hurt you every now and then.

3. *Dinner Out*. I love to eat out. People who are watching their weight often think they can't because the temptations will be too great or the restaurant won't have the right foods for them. I have two things to say to these people:

- Phooey
- Phooey

I don't suggest you eat out every night; nor do I propose you go wild, or even pick Mexican when you could be happy eating Japanese. But if you are in a bad mood, or cannot stand the thought of cooking one more meal, or need a psychological break from routine, a dinner out will do you a world of good.

There is one other way to make dinner preparation easier, but it takes advance planning and careful coordination: a dinner co-op. If you can get together a group of friends, or neighbors, who are interested in the same calorie budget as you and your family, you can car-pool your meals. Planned on a five-day-a-week schedule (weekends are free), if you get four other families to join in, each person would be responsible for cooking enough food for the group once a week. The other nights she would not cook at all.

Dinner at a Restaurant

While you are on the Sneaky Plan, it's best to avoid restaurants entirely or to choose only those where you know ahead of time what his choices will be (sushi bars, seafood restaurants, salad bars, etcetera). If you cannot avoid the wrong choice without blowing your cover, just keep your mouth shut and hope he doesn't eat everything in sight.

Aside from the secret part of the food plan, I recommend that each couple eat dinner out once a week if they can afford it. It need not be a ten-course meal at Lutece. It can even be at a pizza parlor—but not every week. Eating dinner out breaks up the week and offers a reward. No matter how strict your food plan, you can always eat out.

There are two safe ways to approach dinner at a restaurant:

1. You alert your husband ahead of time that you're going out, so he can horde a few extra calories. If you've got your man on a 2,000-calorie-a-day budget, he can be very happy having a 500-calorie breakfast, a 500-calorie lunch and a 1,000-calorie dinner. Normally I would prefer the heavier meal at lunch, but, hey, once a week is okay. Besides, after dinner you can walk

around or do something to burn off a few of those calories before you hit the sack.

2. You can help your husband make a priority rating of the menu and come up with the appropriate dish. The average menu will have half a dozen choices within his calorie budget without your asking for anything special.

In the course of solving my husband's weight problem, we have experimented with several restaurants and have developed a list of safe places so that if we want a relaxing meal without any guessing games, we know precisely where to go and what can be ordered.

Going to a restaurant should not cause panic, even if your husband eats lunch out every day. There are enough restaurants that grill fish, serve fresh veggies, and take pride in their salads for you to survive comfortably in the world of menus. Most Italian and Mexican restaurants offer light dishes along with the sybaritic. Check out other ethnic foods also. Our current favorite is Thai food. Read restaurant reviews and guide books for tips. Investigate "diet" restaurants— big cities often have places that provide the calorie counts on the menu along with the meals. Hunt around; seek and ye shall find, and all that.

Dinner at Someone's Home

A person who is on a strict diet feels panic-stricken when invited to a friend's home for dinner. Yes, he is thrilled to be invited; but no, he doesn't want to go because of the fear that when food is placed in front of him, he will lose control, wolf it all down, and blow his food plan. Furthermore, he doesn't know how to tell the hostess that he is watching his weight.

I don't know how often you eat at someone else's house (other than on holidays) or how often you have people to yours, but when you are watching someone else's weight for him, it is a bit easier for you to say something about food choices. When accepting a dinner invitation, or even when planning dinner out with another couple, I always start off the conversation with the limits that are on Mike's diet—"Mike's eating lightly" I say, as coyly as possible. "We'd prefer not to eat meat," or, "Let's try that new seafood restaurant"; these comments often get the point across. Or you can do the ultimate turn-around—if you are invited to friends for dinner, suggest instead that the friends come to you.

It is much easier for wives to get together and protect their husbands than it is for the men to protect themselves. And it is usually best for the plotting to be done out of earshot of the men—husbands do not like to think that their wives control or manipulate their lives, or that anyone is thinking about their weight or special dietary needs. Men do not want anyone to make a big deal of their weight problems! So don't get caught at it. And remember, if it's just an occasional evening out (once every two to three months is occasional), treat it as a holiday—ignore it. Let him eat whatever he's going to eat and worry about taking off the excess *later*.

If you belong to a supper club, get the cooks together and convert them to your calorie budget. It will be good for everyone. Don't be shy. My friend Leah accepted a dinner invitation, then agonized over it so much she decided to cancel. Finally she confessed to the hostess that she had her husband on a special food plan. To her delight, the hostess announced that her husband was on the Pritikin Plan. No one could have been more understanding. *Speak up*—most people have the same problems you do!

7

SPECIAL OCCASIONS

Special Occasion Psychology

To a person who likes food, every day has at least one special occasion, which can make every diet a rope that's just too perilous to walk. It's not hard to come up with an excuse to eat that one special little thing that blows the whole budget. Since this diet is more like Big Brother Is Watching than Dr. Pritikin Is Saying No-No, it's important that the dieter—that's your husband—be allowed his special occasions while still being able to lose weight.

Obviously every day can't be a special occasion, but if your husband thinks he *can't* indulge, he may reject the diet totally. This is why I've asked you to make dinner as festive as possible— it's a psychological maneuver to make your man happier. He will still need to know it's okay sometimes to eat the foods that give him the emotional sustenance he needs. And he'll need traditional holiday foods at the appropriate times. He should *never* feel deprived.

With a 2,000-calorie-a-day budget, he cannot

have an extra treat every day. But once a week won't kill him. Ignore it when he slips up. No matter what he does, remind him you still love him and believe in him and his ability to take off weight. If he persistently overdoes it, he may need a little professional guidance. That's not my department, and probably not yours. There are, however, psychologists who specialize in over-eaters; perhaps you can find one in your city.

Wife Trauma

You will suffer wife trauma every time your man goes on an eating binge. Just don't let him know what you're going through. My husband had a self-destructive fling that lasted for three days during which he ate everything in sight and con-vinced me he was experiencing a severe death wish. He never confided his real problem to me. On the fourth day he was back to normal and set about losing the weight he had gained.

No matter how much you do for him, you can't do everything. There will be times you will want to pull your hair out. It's a fact of life.

Oops

In the first two-week period, while the diet is still secret, he won't know when he slips up because he won't know he's *on* a special diet. Keep quiet when he binges, but try to figure why he's doing it.

Once he knows that you're watching his weight, you can police the scene a little more easily, but he may test you, so beware. Allow him one "oops" a week. Beyond that, say something. If you have to mention it a lot, ask if he's really serious about losing weight. If he isn't, return this book before it's too late. If he's serious, he'll thank you for reminding him not to overeat.

To me, an oops is different from a binge. An oops is a one-time, one-item slip of the lip that costs 250 to 500 calories. A binge is an all-out, item-after-item debauch that could add up to several thousand calories. Binges have a detrimental psychological effect on husband and wife; "oopses" do not.

If you go out for drinks, in itself a splurge, and your husband then proceeds to eat all the guacamole dip—that's an oops.

If your child decides he can't finish his praline maple crepe (a la mode) and rather than let it go to waste, your husband decides to clean the plate —that's an oops.

An oops does not happen on a special occasion, because you know about most of them ahead of time and can more or less budget them into your day. An oops is often a mistake or a forgotten priority, rather than a blatant attempt to eat something forbidden. An oops can be worked off by exercise, or simply forgotten. As long as it doesn't happen too often, it's unimportant.

Binges Are Not Special Occasions

A binge is also a mistake, but is usually a deliberate one and has little to do with hunger. A binge is a direct assault on misery but has the unhappy effect of making the perpetrator feel *more* miserable once it's over. Most bingers feel such terrible guilt and anxiety *after* the binge is over that they whip themselves into a frenzy of angst. Most bingers go on a binge as a form of self-punishment or self-loathing. I once read that the average binge accounts for 10,000 calories!

As far as I'm concerned, any adult who is eating more than 2,000 calories a day (who is not in training for the Olympics) has no shortage of food to complain about. He or she won't see it that way, which is, of course, part of the problem. For a man, a binge may be an emotional response to a problem in his life. Or it may hinge on a silly excuse—"I'm on the road; I can't watch my weight," or, "It's a business lunch, I can't just have a piece of fish," and so forth—that gives the man permission to eat what he wants. For the person who comes up with one excuse after another, a binge is a way of life . . . and death.

A binge is a siege of compulsive eating, during which the devil forces one to eat either a particular type of food—chocolate, pasta, cookies, ice cream, cheesecake—or everything in sight. It has *nothing* to do with hunger. Usually the worst bingers are people who keep a preternaturally tight rein on their food plans and forbid themselves to eat "fattening" foods—which is why most bingers are women.

If you see your husband verging on a binge (to avoid disappointing you or hurting your feelings, he will probably try to keep it secret from you; so your in-office spy may be able to help you spot approaching binges), try to find out what has caused it. If it's a one-day binge and then he's back to normal, maybe you can talk *around* the binge and go for what's really on his mind. If he obsesses about certain foods he wants to eat, let him eat them. Denying him will make matters worse. Tension often makes an eater more "hungry." If the binge pattern suddenly appears and does not abate, see if you can get him to keep a food chart. Or see a psychologist. Break him out of the binge slowly and carefully by being loving and reassuring—by giving him permission, not by taking away food. Most men aren't too good at talking about their feelings or their problems; overeating is sometimes their way of admitting they *have* a problem. See if some special effort on your part can get your man to share his pain rather than to hide it under hot fudge. Hugs, sex, presents, and attention can often counteract a binge.

Remember to take it slowly and to be understanding. This is not a time for demands, ultimatums, or scene-staging.

His Special Days

Everybody has days that are special, during which he or she has no interest in being denied anything—especially food. On these days, no man wants to think about what should or shouldn't be eaten. He just wants to relax and eat whatever appeals to him. So on his special days —birthday, Father's Day, perhaps a wedding anniversary, the day a child is born—let him alone. Totally. Chances are he won't stray more than 500 calories over his setpoint anyway. Five hundred extra calories a few days a year are not going to hurt anyone. Even if he eats 1,000 extra calories, it's simply not the end of the world.

As an experiment, I gave my husband several "free" days to gauge the impact on his eating patterns and his weight. Once his setpoint had been changed and he was maintaining 206 pounds, he was quite picky about what he ate even on free days. He *knew* he would gain weight if he went nuts, so he was careful. His over-budget treats were either ice cream, Mexican food, or a margarita or two. That's it. And nothing happened to him—he didn't gain weight, he didn't return to his former eating habits, he didn't feel psychological pangs of guilt or resentment.

Men usually choose to celebrate their special days with nostalgia—a piece of comfort out of their eating past—a drink or two, a piece of cake or pie, ice cream, pasta, or four hot dogs (with buns and loaded with mustard and relish) at the ball game with beer, popcorn, and a chocolate-covered banana on a stick. A special day is sort of like a binge with tradition behind it. Don't deny him!

Other People's Special Days

While it's just fine for him to celebrate his own special days, that's the end of my generosity. Other people's special days are for other people. He's either going to have a few bites over his budget and walk away, or else just say, "No, thank you." If your man celebrates every special occasion that comes his way, he'll look like Santa Claus in no time at all.

If it's your birthday, make it easier on him. Don't have a cake. Have a dessert, either at home or out, that is served in portions. Or share one piece of cake or dessert with him. Go out to lunch and indulge if you want to, but don't put temptation in his way. And don't put your ego on the line and expect him to eat something extra to please *you* on your special day. Have a sorbet with a candle in it; or a scoop of ice cream if you must. But do everyone in the family a favor—don't order butter cream roses and creamy salutations that will only clog the arteries and add inches to the thighs.

Snacks As Special Occasions

Sometimes a snack is a special occasion and should be treated as such.

The Coffee Break. A coffee break serves many important purposes. It can be very awkward for a man to refuse coffee or a doughnut, but with reprogramming your man will learn to accept *only* the coffee and nurse it. If the coffee break is merely a means of escaping work for twenty minutes, it is easier to eliminate. Get your husband's secretary to tell you his coffee break habits, then alter them if possible.

Cocktail Hour. The cocktail hour can be an important adjunct to your husband's business day and as such cannot be dropped from his schedule. However, what he eats and drinks during that hour can indeed be modified. There has already been a big shift away from hard liquor and toward wine or "light" drinks—wine spritzers, sparkling wines, sparkling waters, etcetera. There's a very good reason: Hard liquor is *very* fattening—to say nothing of dangerous when consumed in quantity, particularly before driving home. Men who make the switch from two glasses of scotch to two wine spritzers will enjoy an automatic weight loss. Those who stop nibbling the cocktail snacks will lose even more weight. If a cocktail is part of your husband's daily after-work ritual, it will be almost impossible to have him go without. The cocktail hour serves as an important psychological cushion in bridging the time between office and home. Cocktail hour in your own home can be more easily controlled: serve low-calorie nibbles if they must be served at all, or provide a soup that will actually help fill him up before the meal.

Remind him that cocktails are a special occasion now. Suggest that he volunteer to make the switch away from hard liquor and limit his own drinking. If your husband is a heavy drinker who cannot cut back to two drinks, his overeating and overdrinking may stem from a problem with which an expert can better deal. Light to average drinkers will be able to stay within two drinks per day when they understand the difference it makes in their weight control.

Get these calorie counts:

beer	95
Bloody Mary	140
martini, gin, or vodka, 2 ounces	100
red wine	95
screwdriver, 8 ounces total drink	168
scotch, 2 ounces	130
Tom Collins, 8 ounces total drink	170
whiskey sour	142
white wine	90

After school. The after-school snack has translated into an afternoon coffee break for most of us who feel we deserve a pick-me-up at about 4 P.M. For kids who need calories, this is an ideal time to feed them the extra food that will not be on the table when Dad comes home. For people who are watching their weight, this snack period should be eliminated or reduced to a cup of herb tea, iced tea, water, or at most, a piece of fruit. Men who go out for cocktails rarely have four o'clock breaks, but men who work longer hours and know they won't be leaving the office until six-thirty or seven usually tell themselves they "deserve" or "need" this fuel supply time.

Bedtime. Bedtime is a favorite snack time because it is associated with childhood. You can almost hear Mom's voice and smell her perfume when you remember the snack she provided before tucking you in. There is little reason for anyone to eat a bedtime snack, even children, so eliminate this habit in your own home now, so that your kids will not grow up with the same problem. Most adults feel sneaky about a bedtime snack—probably because they *know* they don't need it. I've noticed that my husband waits until I'm asleep before slipping downstairs for his snack; in the morning, I find the remnants on his night table. Nowadays, though, I find the remains of an apple core—I used to find a small plate with an occasional chocolate crumb or two.

If your husband does not consider a bedtime treat a special occasion, change his food plan accordingly.

On the Road

For some people, being on the road is a way of life. For others, a business trip is a special occasion. Whatever the situation, most people consider being on the road a good excuse to eat without observing calorie budgets.

Wrong.

If your husband travels a lot, no doubt he has put on weight from the combination of driving all day and stopping at fast-food restaurants, or from getting on planes and eating their heavy foods, from ordering up room service, from having to eat big meals with clients, from keeping long hours and getting no exercise. If you do not travel with your husband, and few wives do, it is going to be difficult to manage his weight from afar. The best you can do is teach him food priorities; the rest is up to him. It may help if you go out with him for a day or two (often airlines have promotional fares allowing wives to fly for half-price or free) and show him how to take care of himself, or on your next vacation, teach him the survival ropes. Maybe only exercise will save him.

- Order low-calorie airline food for him, or ask his secretary to do so. Don't let him eat the standard meal.
- Help him to overcome the loneliness that may lead to overeating: Buy him an absorbing book, perhaps, or arrange for him to be with friends or clients he likes rather than alone.
- Teach him the priority ratings and how to read a menu, so he can cope with all the restaurant food he will encounter.

- Subscribe to one of those national or international health club plans, or only book him (or have his secretary book him) into hotels with health clubs. While a non-traveling husband can lose weight without exercise, your traveling man may need a workout.

Vacations

For most people, a vacation is a chance to go off a food plan. My plan is so liberal that he doesn't know he's "on" it, so hopefully he won't need to go "off" it. Therefore, a trip can be treated as a special occasion and forgotten . . . especially if it's five to seven days long. (For longer periods, he's *got* to be careful.)

We went on a New Mexican holiday that included lots of Mexican food, afternoon strolls munching on ice cream cones, and a few extra steak dinners. At the end of five days of eating everything he wanted, Mike gained a total of two pounds. He was able to lose them in less than two weeks. No big deal, and a good time was had by all.

Then, we returned to New Mexico for a ski trip. Disaster. There were only two grocery stores at our ski resort, both with a slender selection of fresh foods—limited produce, only three or four types of meat, no fish. We were forced to use canned goods and frozen foods, to eat beef. It was virtually impossible to fix a week's worth of faux gourmet meals. Mike gained six pounds in five days—and it wasn't even *fun*.

So my advice about vacations is simple: Enjoy

them, but spend them in big cities or areas where you know you can get fresh foods.

• You can choose between ten different meal choices on your vacation flight, as long as you put your order in at least twenty-four hours before takeoff. Ask for the choices and the calorie count on each. Usually, there is a low-calorie meal, a low-sodium meal, a kosher meal, a seafood meal, a fruit tray, a vegetarian meal, etcetera. The average airplane meal is 800 calories and not very nutritious. Bring your own meal or order a 500-calorie version. Sometimes the low-cal meal has more calories than the fruit tray, so ask.

• Eating lightly in the air fights jet lag and won't hurt your figure.

• During the flight, drink lots of liquids, but *no* alcoholic drinks and preferably no soft drinks. Avoid spicy foods, sugar, and salt. (Give back the free peanuts—you don't really want them!) Eating lightly does not mean skipping meals.

• Try to stick to three meals a day eaten at regular meal times. The more snacking you do, the more weight you'll gain. If you need an afternoon break to rest your feet, have fruit if possible, because it offers natural rather than refined sugar.

• Drink lots of water during your vacation.

• Check out the local dishes, especially if your vacation is in a foreign country. If they are fried, dipped in batter, sugary, or salty—avoid them. If they are fresh, natural, light, and still tasty— enjoy. If you try a national dish that turns out to be covered in sauce, gravy, or cream, pick out the chunks without sopping up the sauce. Avoid raw foods and tap water in some foreign countries. Fresh fruits that can be peeled or husked are okay.

• Lay off the bread products, no matter how good.

• Stop at grocery stores and outdoor markets for fresh foods, rather than at roadside restaurants or greasy spoons. A rotisserie chicken, some carefully chosen cheese (Laughing Cow makes a reduced-calorie cheese that is only 35 calories per three-quarter-ounce triangle), and fresh fruit will make a much better meal than one eaten at a fast-food restaurant. It's no harder to get off the freeway to stop at a supermarket than it is to get to a restaurant. Most major cities in America (and around the world for that matter) have markets that are tourist attractions—pay them a visit and enjoy.

More and more, there are vacation spots that advertise low-calorie fare, exercise programs, and overall health benefits. There is a Club Med vacation where a doctor will check you out and tell you exactly what to eat. There are sports-oriented vacations: tennis camps, rafting trips, climbing trips, trekking, and so forth. You can get away from it all, have a great time, and come home thin.

Holidays

In most cultures, holidays mean food. Luckily for your husband, holidays are not as hard on men as they are on women. (Faced with most of the food preparation, women tend to eat more during the holidays.) Your husband can enjoy himself and still have a very merry if you both remember these rules:

• Pass on alcoholic drinks whenever possible. If he insists on drinking, have wine or better yet, lite wine. Champagne also comes in a lite version. A glass of champagne is always to be preferred to a glass of eggnog and rum, or to a scotch and soda. No matter how dismal the office Christmas party, don't get bombed! He'll easily consume 1,000 calories getting drunk—maybe more—and could eat another 1,000 to 3,000 in snacks and junk.

• Make choices. Choose bread or stuffing, not both.

• If both ham and turkey are served, go heavier on the turkey—it's much less fatty. You don't have to bypass the ham totally, but two slices of turkey to one slice of ham is the wiser ratio. (Remove skin from turkey; fat from ham.)

• Do not have seconds.

• Don't bring food as gifts and ask your friends to refrain as well.

• Don't serve (or eat) salted snack foods or candy.

• Don't eat everything on your plate. Remember your children and how much they need you. Aim to eat half of everything on your plate.

• Try to eat meals at regular meal times rather than at crazy hours.

• Pass up whatever sweets may be associated with the holiday, but eat dessert after the big holiday meal. No, he doesn't need that chocolate rabbit.

• Never mention in the course of the meal or during any of the festivities that you or your husband are "watching your weight."

- If you are the hostess, give away the party leftovers.
- If you are the guest, don't volunteer to help in the kitchen. Stay away from food plates (or keep your husband away), including dirty dishes.
- Eat a healthy meal before going to a party; never arrive hungry. Never tell your man you don't feel like cooking and that he should "make a meal" from the snacks.
- If there is dancing, football, or any kind of physical activity attached to the holiday celebration, encourage your husband to participate.
- Don't wear clothes that are too loose to the party. Tight clothes that will be uncomfortable are unnecessary, but avoid wearing "fat clothes" to enable you to eat plenty of food. It's a bad psychological move that guarantees overeating.

Since holidays are usually family affairs, prepare yourself psychologically beforehand. You or your husband will witness old eating habits, will hear the same relatives begging you to eat, will see and smell dishes that conjure up powerful memories; you may even be sitting in the chair you graced as a child. It will be a lot harder than usual for either of you to be strong. Family reunions can also cause tension; tension causes many people to overeat. Give yourself some leeway and then fight silently for the rest of your dignity. If you see your husband revert to his childhood, do not mention it. When you are back home, or after the company has left, return to a strict calorie budget and fight whatever weight gain may have ensued over the holiday.

Remember: Holidays are not happy occasions for everyone—if depression or anxiety make your husband indulge, try some modification in your

153

holiday plans. Maybe this is the year you don't go to grandmother's house after all.

Having It All

The key to having your special occasions and keeping your figure is to do all things in moderation. Hardly a radical thought, but an important one. Your husband should be able to eat some birthday cake, toss down a few beers when his team takes the Series or on Superbowl Sunday, go out to dinner, go on vacation—lead a perfectly normal life without gaining weight. He can do all these things, in fact, and keep *losing* weight . . . when he has a wife who keeps his calorie budget intact.

8

EXERCISE

Yes He Can

It is a scientific fact that the best way to lose weight and keep it off is to combine a program of smart eating with serious exercise.

It is *also* a scientific fact that you can lose weight *without* exercising at all. Especially if you are a man.

While I recommend that every person in the world exercise regularly and get a nice combination of aerobic, stretching, and endurance exercises, I can recommend until I'm blue in the face. That doesn't get you, or your husband, onto the stationary bicycle (I know you've got one in your garage; we do too) or onto the exercise mat. While you *can* control a good bit of what your husband eats, you *cannot* do leg lifts for him.

So don't try.

Modern exercise gurus aside, there are still many people who really don't *want* to exercise. I would gladly forgo dessert not to have to go to exercise class. Millions of people feel the same.

If your husband eats 500 fewer calories per

day, he should *automatically* (without exercise) lose one pound a week.

If he eats 1,000 fewer calories per day, he should *automatically* (without exercise) lose two pounds a week.

Once he establishes a new setpoint for his body, he will find the proper calorie budget for comfort and satisfaction, and he will maintain his weight loss. He will only *gain* weight if he increases his calorie intake.

If he does endurance exercises, he will either lose more weight or be able to increase his calorie budget accordingly. If he does aerobic exercises, he will make his heart and lungs work better but will probably not lose much weight.

In a combined exercise and reduced-calorie budget, a man can eat 250 fewer calories and exercise off an additional 250 calories (one hour of bowling will do it) to take off the same amount of weight that will automatically come off by reducing food intake by 500 calories. My husband would rather go without a dessert than go to the gym. As much as I talk about going bowling, we never do. He could burn off 250 calories by pushing a power mower around the yard for one hour, but our yard is covered with ivy. He could lose 210 calories by biking at 5½ mph for an hour, but he won't do that either. His is a very sedentary life-style. Giving up food is easier for him than taking on Tarzan. Some husbands are jocks, obsessed with their muscles. Mine is not. Yet that hasn't stopped him from losing and keeping off a big hunk of weight.

Old-Fashioned Theories

In the old days, about twenty or thirty years ago, few doctors recommended exercise in conjunction with diet as a method of weight loss. They were wrong, but you have to examine the rationale behind the theory: Doctors felt it would be discouraging to patients if they realized exactly how much exercise was needed to take off weight! This was way before the current fitness boom and Jack LaLanne was at that time the only healthy man in America. Designer leotards had not yet been invented, jogging was not the rage —and you got athlete's foot at a gym.

Doctors instead suggested that their patients play a little golf or tennis and follow a sensible food plan, much like the one outlined in this book. They always stressed eating less, rather than exercising more. And people who followed their doctors' suggestions lost weight. Without exercise.

New research has provided a multitude of impressive reasons why everyone should exercise. But this does not mean that the old-fashioned way won't work.

The Facts About Exercise and Weight Loss

Exercise burns up calories. The reduction of calories results in weight loss. That's why active teenage boys and professional athletes can eat thousands of calories and not put on weight. That's why inactive middle-aged men gain.

Unfortunately, most of us are not athletes. White-collar husbands sit at desks most of the day, getting little or no exercise. (Blue-collar husbands do get more exercise, true, but that doesn't mean they are in good shape.) While there are many corporate programs that reward executives for losing weight, exercising, quitting smoking, jogging, etcetera, the average AH (American Husband) is not offered an incentive by his company, has no free gym facilities, does not take the time for a regular exercise program, and may or may not be involved in a weekend sport. He may have been a jock in high school; he may consider himself merely "out of shape." He probably wishes he "had the time" to exercise and even realizes that the lack of exercise is bad for his health. Yet he does little about it. Exercising is not a top priority. The average AH has his hands full just getting by. He may even think that plopping down on the sofa with a few beers and watching Monday night football is his due after a hard day's work. He does not want to know from fitness.

For women, exercise is a vital part of the weight loss process because it is so much harder for them to lose weight and keep it off. For men, as much as they may *need* the exercise, a good workout is not crucial to their ability to lose or keep off weight. (No one said life was going to be fair.)

A recent research study at the University of California at Davis compared weight loss of three different groups of dieters. The first group reduced daily food intake by 500 calories; the second increased physical activity to burn off an additional 500 calories a day; and the third group ate 250 fewer calories and increased activity to burn off 250 calories. The weight loss was similar in all three groups, *but* the group that dieted *without exercise* did not lose as much body fat as the others.

If you are trying to do a complete renovation on your husband's body, he will need to exercise for an hour at least four times a week. That's not impossible, and you can offer Sneaky Exercise as an alternative (see page 169). But you can still get twenty pounds off your man, and thereby increase the length of his life, without an exercise program. Honest Injun.

He Ain't Heavy, He's My Hubby

If your husband is grossly overweight, do not advise him to exercise without a doctor's approval. Your doctor will probably advise that you take the twenty pounds off him first, *then* help him to begin a slow but steady fitness regimen along with a continued plan of sensible calorie budgeting.

Grossly overweight people should go especially easy on aerobic exercise, and must have their doctor's approval. If your man is fifty or more pounds overweight, consult your doctor. Period.

Exercise and Calorie Counting

How much weight can your AH expect to burn off if he gets off his duff? Here's a list of activities with the number of calories burned **if** he does the exercise for **one hour**:

Walking, 2½ mph . . . 210 calories **per hour**
Walking, 3¾ mph . . . 300 calories **per hour**
Biking, 5½ mph . . . 210 calories **per hour**
Biking, 13 mph . . . 660 calories **per hour**
Gardening . . . 220 calories **per hour**
Golfing . . . 250 calories **per hour**
Bowling . . . 270 calories **per hour**
Tennis . . . 420 calories **per hour**
Swimming . . . 720 calories **per hour**
Running, 10 mph . . . 900 calories **per hour**
Chopping wood . . . 400 calories **per hour**
Cross-country skiing . . . 500 calories **per hour**
Sex . . . 150 calories PER HOUR

As you can see, the amount of exercise needed for a small loss is not especially encouraging. Sure, there are sneaky exercise and sports your man will enjoy. Great. But, unless he's a dedicated jock, you will probably have trouble getting him to commit to an army training program. Look at the numbers above and relax! It may not be worth the nagging. And get this, Dr. Jere Mitchell at Southwestern Medical School in Dallas notes that in a study of cross-country skiers in Scandinavia, increased life span was only two years. "That's not enough of a benefit to most people," he notes.

Fighting Flabola

Because of the body fat distribution in a man's body, men usually get pot bellies and love handles. When they lose weight, they lose in these areas first. If your husband loses twenty pounds on this food plan and does not exercise, will he turn to mush?

Probably not. Maybe, but probably not. My husband didn't. My husband lost a total of 37 pounds without exercise: He lost one chin and his love handles, and was miraculously rewarded with a flat stomach. He was forced both to put little green dots on his size 38 belts (blue dots on the size 40's) and to buy a whole new wardrobe. He even bought several pairs of *pleated* trousers.

The rate at which stretched-out skin resembles flab depends on each person's body. Exercise will definitely help, but if there is a dramatic weight loss, a plastic surgeon just might need to nip and tuck.

This is an individual matter that requires a wait-and-see approach.

Heart and Soul

As the caretaker of my husband's health, I am more concerned that he have aerobic exercise than exercise to lose weight, reshape his body, or become as supple as a Kleenex. It's his heart and lungs that I want in prime condition. After all, the purpose of the diet is to take the strain off of them so the big body beautiful can keep on glowing.

Fifteen minutes of aerobic exercise three times a week *combined* with a loss of twenty pounds will indeed improve your husband's life and future.

While aerobic exercise for women has become quite the thing, with dance classes and self-defense classes popping up in every neighborhood, a man does not need to go to class (neither does a woman for that matter) in order to strengthen his heart.

The word "aerobic" was popularized by Dr. Kenneth Cooper; it means "with oxygen." Aerobic exercise is rhythmic repetitive exercise that increases the body's ability to deliver blood—with its oxygen and nourishment—to the muscles and organs. The best aerobic exercises are the ones that produce a high heart rate and demand a large amount of oxygen. As you build up your endurance for the aerobic activity, your heart and lungs are strengthened and actually function better.

Aerobic Exercise

Aerobic exercise is dynamic and requires constant movement without rest. Restive exercise (a game of golf or a ten-second sprint across the yard) is called anaerobic and may burn calories but does little to improve the performance of the cardiovascular system. Walking, jogging, swimming, running, race-walking, cycling (free or stationary bike), skipping rope, and cross-country skiing are good aerobic exercises.

Aerobic exercise makes the major muscle groups work harder and, at the same time, frees arteries and veins from blockages. If your husband is chubby or has had a diet of junk foods and fatty foods, he needs a good bit of unclogging.

For the person who is unused to any activity, aerobic exercise should be begun slowly and then built up to a fifteen-minute period. A warm-up and cool-down are also vital. During the warm-up, the body temperature rises and the increased need for oxygen in the newly exerted muscles makes the heart beat faster. If your husband jumps too fast into too much exercise, he could have a heart attack. If he does not warm up muscles, he can damage them. The warm-up gets the blood flowing and the body ready for the aerobic routine.

He can warm up using a videotape, his own exercise program, or any number of celebrity-inspired methods. Since we're not too big on exercise in our house, we use the lazy man's warm-up: five minutes of riding the stationary bicycle at a slow speed—about 5 to 7 mph. Then we rev up to 15 mph for another ten minutes. That's all folks, that's the whole work-out. It does nothing for the arms, it does not increase the size of the chest nor does it reduce backache. *But,* it does work out the heart. (Yes, it's also good for the legs.) It will help prolong our lives—if we're careful crossing streets and don't meet up with any deranged snipers. For people like Mike and me, fifteen minutes on the bike is the best we can do.

If your husband is in the same boat as mine—slightly overweight (even with the twenty-pound loss), inactive, a family history of heart trouble—the most important kind of exercise he can get is aerobic. There are easy ways of getting it. The simplest aerobic exercises for men, ones that can be performed right there at home with little extra equipment and no need for special clothing, are

- riding the stationary bicycle
- jumping rope
- using a treadmill or running machine
- jogging up and down the stairs

- using a rowing machine
- swimming (if you have a pool)
- jogging in place

To get him going, help organize the daily schedule so that there is *time* for these events. His biggest excuse for not exercising will be that he's too busy. If you, or other family members (when age and talent permit), join in and make exercise time a must-do family fun time, you will be able to establish one of your family's most important health habits.

Knowing how important exercise could be to Mike's life, but unable to get him—or myself—motivated, made me ashamed, disgusted, and embarrassed. Yet none of these are aerobic responses. I was *determined* to come up with some way to make him exercise without standing over him, whip in hand. Knowing the stationary bicycle was still our best bet, I dragged old faithful out of the garage, dusted it off, and drove to Sears where I bought a second stationary bicycle. I placed both of them in front of the television set, and announced we would do this the same way we lost the weight—together.

Endurance Exercise

Endurance exercise is pumping iron—it can make you muscular and strong and can rebuild or reshape your body. It works up a sweat, and, depending on your physical goals, can take hours a day. While it is the type of exercise that helps you control your weight or rearrange your inches, it is also time-consuming. It's a great anti-depressant, it gives you tons of energy, it's fabulous for your body and, in theory, I recommend it to everyone. It's just got one thing wrong with it—you have to do it. Many people, men and women, can't find the time or the motivation.

Endurance exercise provides flexibility, strength, and—you guessed it—endurance. Most men can exert themselves for a short period of time: to run after the bus, to pick up a suitcase for a lady, to carry the fifty-pound sack of sand from the car to the sandbox. If the body is out of shape, these activities may cause pain, even injury, and cannot be sustained for more than a few minutes. Hard labor and constant muscular workout are the only things that give you the ability to take these tasks lightly. Your husband will still get winded when he races your son across the yard, or still complain about the weight of your grocery bags, unless he has a program of endurance exercises, which have nothing to do with sports or aerobic exercise. Riding that stationary bike each morning will *not* make the groceries any lighter!

Stretching

The third type of exercise is stretching, another way to add flexibility to the body. Stretching is fabulous for eliminating tension, revving up circulation, and making you come back to life after sitting around. It does not take weight off, nor is it an aerobic exercise.

Stretching is a good warm-up to aerobics and is a great way to start the day. It's also particularly good for people with back trouble.

My husband does a series of stretches each

morning and night only because he has a trick back that seems to respect stretching. The morning stretches also serve as a warm-up to his biking.

Sports

Most men think sports are the same as exercise. They are not.

You exercise certain muscles performing various sports activities. While swimming is a great overall sport, most sports use a particular set of muscles and that's it. A sport may be a great way of working up a sweat and even jettisoning some calories, but when performed only on an occasional or weekend basis, it doesn't accomplish anything near what He-Man thinks it does.

Sports are great for releasing tension, working off aggression, strengthening friendships, and creating team spirit. They are not the answer to your husband's need for aerobic exercise—unless his sport happens to be one of the aerobic fitness sports and he performs it for fifteen minutes or more several times a week.

The man who swims or plays tennis every day or every other day is probably in good shape. Bless his heart, it will beat forever and make his wife happy. The man who has no regular daily activity at all and who plays a game of touch football with the guys one weekend or hits balls with his son on a Saturday afternoon is not going to burn off many calories, give his heart any kind of regular workout, or improve his body to prolong his life. He may even hurt himself; since weekend athletes, usually in bad shape, have the most injuries.

While sports should be enjoyed for the pure physical activity involved, they must be played with regularity to be of a life-prolonging nature. The man who regularly jogs, rides a bike, kayaks, hikes, swims laps, plays one-on-one, is part of a regular soccer team with practice and games, or plays racquetball or tennis religiously—participating in this sort of activity for about an hour at least three times a week—has done something to help himself and his body. The AH cannot count his sports activities as any form of anatomical resuscitation.

If you have kids who are old enough to play sports, or have social plans with other couples whose sporting talents are similar (in playing, not in watching), you can encourage your husband to make social (and business) connections through sports. If this isn't your style (my major sporting activity is shopping), concentrate on his aerobic program and forget the rest.

The Lazy Man's Exercise Trick

If your husband has no interest in sports, if you can't get him onto that stationary bike, if all your nagging, pleading, social scheduling, and clever ideas have not gotten him out of his arm chair in front of the television set, I have one last ace up my sleeve. Walking.

Most men do not consider walking a sport, so you can trick them into it. To develop and maintain a healthy body, the average person (man or woman) should walk a brisk 3½ miles per hour. This is not browsing-around-the-mall pace, nor is it running the four-minute mile. You need to walk for at least half an hour; forty or fifty minutes is better. You will burn calories if you walk at a brisk pace (slower doesn't count), and you will give your heart and lungs the aerobic exercise they need. Furthermore, it's a good partner sport for a husband and wife (or the whole family) and gives you some time together. Even if you can't talk while you're walking that fast (you can, but it hurts), you can be together, commune with nature, and hold hands.

Some other ways to get a little walking in:

- Park the car far from the market or the shopping center and walk to the stores. Yes, he'll make a rude comment to you, but he'll walk.
- Go for an after-dinner stroll, be it around your neighborhood, around the high school track, or at a shopping mall. This need not be at 3½ mph; slower will aid digestion and give you some peaceful time together. Remember, this is no longer an aerobic sport, but it's nice nonetheless.
- Encourage him to use the stairs rather than the elevator in his office building. When you go places together, challenge him to take the stairs.

Don't push walking as a sport or health-enhancing maneuver. Merely put on your sensible shoes; then go out and do it. Set up errands that can be walked rather than driven to. Take the time to force yourself—and him with you—to walk a mile or two, hopefully at a nice brisk pace. A brisk walk will keep you from spending and help trim the hips. Be sure to breathe properly if you are planning on talking and walking, otherwise you'll find yourself out of breath quickly or slowing your pace to a crawl. Without getting into race-walking, a popular new sport, use your feet to get you someplace. One mile of brisk walking five or six nights a week (preferably after dinner) will improve both your marriage and your life span.

Sneaky Exercise

There are certain activities that use up calories, are called "exercise" but are really fun—some are sports, some are not. If you can work some of them into your weekly routine, you will both benefit. I don't count the calories they will burn off, because it's meaningless. Anything lost is a benefit, and that's that. Enjoy each other's company (or invite friends along), and enjoy the activity; the burnt-off calories are a bonus:

- Disco dancing
- Break dancing
- Square dancing
- Walking
- Bowling
- Gardening
- Sailing
- Hiking
- Fishing
- Horseback riding
- Skin diving
- Roller skating
- Ping-Pong (table tennis)
- Sex

The Shape of Things to Come

There is a tremendous amount of pressure on people today to be "in shape," which they mistakenly think means thin. You can be thin without being in shape; you can be roundish and in shape. Your husband does not have to be built like Conan the Barbarian to live a long, healthy life.

Your job is not to run your husband's life. If he's interested in being in prime physical condition, that's his business. He probably isn't because he would have never let himself get in the shape he's in now if he really cared. But that's his business. Your business is feeding him low-calorie healthful foods and keeping his weight at a safe level. I know you can mind your own business and help your man to live longer.

CALORIE COUNTS

Whose Counting?

The reason I suggest you use my method of calorie budgeting rather than counting is very simple —I've never been able to find two calorie counters that agree! I've seen martinis listed at 70 calories, 115 calories, and 155 calories! He can either give up his martini totally, or budget it at about 100 and call it a day.

While I have inserted several calorie counts and lists throughout this book, they are merely ball-park figures. These numbers come from hours spent poring over an assortment of books and walking down aisles of grocery stores with a small tape recorder in my hand. If you aim for a 1,500-calorie day, and budget loosely, you'll still be under 2,000 calories—so don't make yourself crazy.

FOOD	QUANTITY	CALORIES
Alcoholic Beverages		
ale	12 ounces	160
beer	12 ounces	160
bourbon	1½ ounces	125
brandy	1½ ounces	75
champagne	4 ounces	85
gin	1½ ounces	110
rum	1½ ounces	100
vodka	1½ ounces	70
whiskey	1½ ounces	105
wines	8 ounces	200

FOOD	QUANTITY	CALORIES
Non-Alcoholic Beverages		
apple juice	4 ounces	60
coffee, black	1 cup	0
cola drinks	8 ounces	96
cranberry juice	8 ounces	130
ginger ale	8 ounces	70
grapefruit juice, fresh	8 ounces	95
frozen concentrate	8 ounces	115
grape juice	8 ounces	160
lemon juice	1 tablespoon	5
lime juice	1 tablespoon	5
orange juice, fresh	8 ounces	110
peach nectar	8 ounces	112
pear nectar	8 ounces	120
pineapple juice	8 ounces	120
prune juice	8 ounces	186
root beer	8 ounces	100
tea	8 ounces	3
tomato juice	6 ounces	32

Dairy Products

<u>Cheese</u>

Camembert	1 ounce	104
cheddar	1 ounce	110
cottage, 2% milkfat	1½ cup	98
cream cheese	1 ounce	105
mozzarella	1 ounce	80
Parmesan	1 tablespoon	24
ricotta, skim milk	4 ounces	85
Romano	1 ounce	110
Roquefort	1 ounce	105
Swiss	1 ounce	100

<u>Eggs</u>

hard boiled	1 large	80
poached	1 large	80
raw, white	1 large	15
yolk	1 large	58

172

FOOD	QUANTITY	CALORIES
scrambled, milk and butter	1 large	112
scrambled, plain	1 large	82

Milk and Cream

butter	1 tablespoon	100
buttermilk	8 ounces	95
evaporated milk	4 ounces	170
half-and-half	4 ounces	162
ice cream, vanilla	½ cup	146
ice milk	½ cup	100
margarine	1 tablespoon	100
sherbet	½ cup	130
skim milk	8 ounces	98
sour cream	4 ounces	240
whipping cream, light	1 tablespoon	45
heavy	1 tablespoon	50
whole milk	8 ounces	160
yogurt	1 cup	115

Vegetables

asparagus	4 spears	12
avocado	½ large	175
beans:		
wax	1 cup	25
green	1 cup	30
lima	½ cup	98
beets, cooked	1 cup	65
broccoli	1 cup	45
cabbage, raw	1 cup	20
cooked	1 cup	27
cabbage, red	1 cup	20
carrots, raw	1 cup	25
cooked	1 cup	35
cauliflower	1 cup	30
celery	1 cup	20
cucumber	1 medium	15
eggplant	1 cup	35
endive	1 cup	10

FOOD	QUANTITY	CALORIES
haricot vert	1 cup	250
leeks	1 cup	100
lettuce	1 cup	10
mushrooms	1 cup	40
okra	1 cup	40
olives, black	1 large	9
green	3 medium	15
onions, raw	1 cup	65
parsley	1 tablespoon	1
parsnip	1 cup	100
peas	1 cup	105
peppers, green	1 medium	15
red	1 medium	20
potatoes:		
baked, plain	1 medium	90
boiled	1 medium	105
mashed, with milk	1 cup	130
radishes	4 small	7
spinach	1 cup	40
sprouts, alfalfa	1 cup	40
squash:		
spaghetti	2 ounces	190
summer	1 cup	25
winter	1 cup	125
sweet potatoes:		
baked	1 medium	150
boiled	1 medium	165
candied	1 medium	290
tomato	1 medium	27
turnips	1 cup	40
watercress	1 cup	8
zucchini	1 cup	50

Fruits

apple	1 medium	80
applesauce, unsweet-ened	1 cup	100
apricots, raw	3 medium	58
banana, raw	1 medium	135
blackberries	1 cup	100

FOOD	QUANTITY	CALORIES
blueberries	1 cup	90
boysenberries	1 cup	65
cantaloupe	½ medium	50
casaba	½ medium	180
cherries, sour	1 cup	100
sweet	1 cup	115
cranberry, canned		
sauce	¼ cup	100
dates	10	230
figs	2 large	60
grapefruit	½ medium	45
grapes	1 cup	100
honeydew	¼ melon	128
kumquats	1 medium	15
lemon	1 medium	20
lime	1 small	20
litchi nuts, fresh	10	60
mangos	1	150
nectarine	1 medium	65
orange	1 medium	75
papaya	½ medium	65
peaches	1 medium	35
pears	1 medium	112
persimmons	1 medium	85
pineapple, fresh	1 cup	80
plums	1 medium	31
pomegranate	1 large	95
prunes	¼ cup	105
raisins	¼ cup	120
raspberries, red	1 cup	70
black	1 cup	100
rhubarb, unsweetened	1 cup	25
strawberries	1 cup	55
tangerine	1 medium	40
watermelon	1 cup	60

Poultry

chicken:		
breast	6 ounces	185
drumstick	6 ounces	200

FOOD	QUANTITY	CALORIES
thigh	6 ounces	200
wing	6 ounces	198
turkey, dark meat	6 ounces	205
light meat	6 ounces	192
veal, average cut	3½ ounces	185
cutlet	3½ ounces	190

Meat

beef:

chuck	6 ounces	280
flank	6 ounces	245
ground beef, lean	4 ounces	212
porterhouse	6 ounces	275
rib roast	6 ounces	330
rump roast	6 ounces	270
sirloin steak	6 ounces	250

lamb:

chop	6 ounces	210
leg	6 ounces	360

liver:

beef	4 ounces	155
calf	4 ounces	155
chicken	4 ounces	146
liver pâté	1 tablespoon	50

pork:

bacon, Canadian	4 ounces	245
chops	4 ounces	266

Breads

breadcrumbs	1 cup	230
cornbread	1 slice	190
cracked wheat	1 slice	63
French	1 slice	57
Italian	1 slice	57
melba toast	1 slice	15
pumpernickel	1 slice	56
raisin	1 slice	60
rye	1 slice	58

FOOD	QUANTITY	CALORIES
white	1 slice	63
whole wheat	1 slice	59

Grains and Cereals

barley	1 cup	700
biscuits	1 2½-inch	135
bran flakes (40%)	1 cup	90
farina	1 cup	100
cornmeal	1 cup	400
oatmeal	1 cup	150
noodles	½ cup	100
pancakes, regular	4-inch diameter	60
buckwheat	1 cake	45
pizza	1 slice (⅛ of pie)	160
popcorn	1 cup	55
rice	1 cup	200
rice, puffed	1 cup	55
spaghetti	1 cup	145
waffles	7-inch diameter	210
wheat, puffed	1 cup	100
wheat, shredded	1 ounce	100
wheat flakes	1 ounce	100
wheat flours:		
all-purpose	1 cup	400
self-rising	1 cup	380
whole wheat	1 cup	420
wheat germ	1 tablespoon	25

Desserts

cakes:

angel food	¹⁄₁₂ of 10-inch cake	130
brownie	2 × 2 × ¾ inch	145
fruitcake	2 × 2 × ½ inch	105
gingerbread	2 × 2 × 2 inch	175
cupcake, plain	1 medium	110
pound cake	½-inch slice	135
sponge cake	¹⁄₁₂ of 10-inch cake	130

FOOD	QUANTITY	CALORIES
candy:		
caramel	1 small piece	35
chocolate cream	1 medium piece	50
gum drop	1 small	10
Lifesaver	1	10
cookies:		
chocolate chip	1 average	50
fig bar	1 square	50
gingersnap	1 small	30
oatmeal	1 large	65
sandwich type	1	50
sugar wafer	1	23
custard	½ cup	150
doughnut	1 medium	125
gelatin	½ cup	70
tapioca	½ cup	110

Seafood

FOOD	QUANTITY	CALORIES
anchovies	3 fillets	21
bass, striped	3½ ounces	100
clams	3½ ounces	76
cod	3½ ounces	170
crab	6 ounces	180
flounder	6 ounces	160
haddock	6 ounces	160
halibut	4½ ounces	230
lobster	6 ounces	190
mussels	3½ ounces	95
ocean perch	6 ounces	160
oysters	4 ounces	80
red snapper	6 ounces	180
salmon, broiled	4 ounces	200
sardines	4 medium	85
scallops	4 ounces	150
seabass	4 ounces	110
shrimp	12–14 medium	100
sole	4 ounces	95
swordfish	4 ounces	130
trout	4 ounces	135

FOOD	QUANTITY	CALORIES
tuna, canned in water	3½ ounces	125
whitefish	4 ounces	165

Specialties and Miscellaneous

FOOD	QUANTITY	CALORIES
bouillon cube	1	4
catsup	1 tablespoon	16
caviar	1 ounce	90
chewing gum	1 stick	10
chocolate syrup	1 tablespoon	48
cocoa	1 tablespoon	20
hollandaise sauce	1 tablespoon	50
honey	1 tablespoon	60
horseradish	1 tablespoon	6
jam	1 tablespoon	55
jelly	1 tablespoon	50
matzoh	1 square	130
mayonnaise	1 tablespoon	100
molasses	1 tablespoon	50
mustard	1 tablespoon	12
peanuts	8–10	55
peanut butter	1 tablespoon	93
pickles	1 medium	10
sauerkraut	½ cup	20
soy sauce	1 tablespoon	12
sugar:		
brown	1 tablespoon	50
	1 cup	800
granulated	1 tablespoon	45
	1 cup	720
powdered	1 tablespoon	30
	1 cup	480
syrup (maple)	1 tablespoon	50
tartar sauce	1 tablespoon	70
vinegar	1 cup	30
yeast	1 package	25

Oils, Fats, and Shortenings

FOOD	QUANTITY	CALORIES
chicken fat	1 tablespoon	125
lard	1 tablespoon	126

FOOD	QUANTITY	CALORIES
salad or cooking oils:		
corn	1 tablespoon	120
cottonseed	1 tablespoon	120
olive	1 tablespoon	118
peanut	1 tablespoon	118
safflower	1 tablespoon	122
sunflower	1 tablespoon	122

FOOD FOR THOUGHT: FAUX GOURMET RECIPES

First, a word from me . . .

There seems to be considerable controversy these days about where recipes come from, since we all know that the stork does not deliver them. The recipes in this book all come from my head, my heart, and my hearth. They have never before been published; many of them are adapted from meals my mother and my grandmother used to make. They are not very grand, but they're not very difficult either. I have not given precise calorie counts, since that is not how this plan works. Each meal is budgeted at 500 calories per person —some run a little more; some, a little less. None is over 600 calories. These are the regular recipes we use in our home; the ones Mike lost weight on. I read in the Framingham Heart Study that the average American household rotates no more than ten dinner recipes throughout the year. In our family, we rotate the ones in this section and eat out one or two nights a week.

Breakfast

We do not have a lot of breakfast recipes, because we eat just about the same thing for breakfast almost every weekday. On weekends, the meals get a little fancier. Mike's Mix (below) can run over 600 calories, but because it's eaten in the morning, it's okay. It's a healthy breakfast and certainly beats bacon and eggs.

MIKE'S MIX

In a very large jar or airtight container, mix equal portions of Crackling Oat Bran, Grape Nuts (not Grape Nut Flakes), All-Bran, and 100% Natural Raisin & Date Cereal. Mix with wooden spoon; store tightly closed. For breakfast serve 6 ounces cereal with low-fat milk or 4 ounces cereal with one sliced banana and low-fat milk. Eliminate raisins to lower caloric intake.

QUICK NUTTY SANDWICH BREAKFAST

1 unsalted rice cake
2 tablespoons crunch-style peanut butter
2 teaspoons low-sugar fruit spread (any flavor)
8 ounces low-fat milk

ALMOST BAGEL AND LOX

1 plain water bagel, split in half
2 tablespoons cream cheese with lox spread

1. After slicing the bagel in half, pull out some of the doughy bread part in the middle and throw it away.
2. Spread one tablespoon of the lox-cream cheese on each half. We buy the lox-cream cheese already prepared at the deli. If you choose to make your own, dice 2 ounces of lox and mix

with 4 ounces whipped cream cheese. Refrigerate remainder. Keeps for about one week.

STRAWBERRY MINI-SHAKE

Serves two.

1 cup fresh strawberries, pureed
1 ice cube
1 8-ounce carton plain, low-fat yogurt
2 eggs (optional)

1. Clean strawberries and puree in blender or food processor.
2. Chop ice cube in food processor.
3. Mix yogurt, strawberry puree, and ice by hand. Add beaten eggs. Stir until well blended.

SPINACH-MUSHROOM OMELET

Serves two.

1 bundle fresh spinach, chopped (1 package frozen, chopped spinach will work)
½ cup sliced, raw mushrooms
Garlic powder to taste
4 eggs
1 scallion, diced

1. Chop fresh spinach. Steam until tender. Set aside.
2. Sauté mushrooms in PAM with garlic. When brown, add spinach. Set aside.
3. Beat eggs with ⅛ cup water and the scallion. Half of the egg mixture combined with half of the spinach mushroom mixture will make each omelet.
4. Spray PAM in medium skillet, add half of

egg mixture (enough for one omelet); when lightly cooked but whole, turn over with spatula.

5. Quickly add half of spinach and mushroom mixture. Then fold half of cooked egg over the mixture. Turn to seal.

BRANCAKES

Serves four.

1¼ cup low-fat milk
1 egg, beaten
1 cup Bisquick
¼ cup unprocessed bran
1 tablespoon cooking oil
4 tablespoons plain low-fat yogurt
1½ cup fresh berries, hulled or sliced

1. Combine milk, egg, Bisquick, and bran. Mix with beaten.
2. Add oil.
3. Spray griddle with PAM, pour batter onto hot griddle.
4. Make small pancakes, so each person can have two.
5. Top each pancake with a tablespoon of yogurt and some berries.

Lunch

We usually go out for lunch, but I have been known to make lunch or to buy appropriate deli foods for serving lunch at home. I often make one of the breakfast recipes (like the omelet or brancakes) for lunch. Lunch is also a good time for a salad.

SUZY'S FAVORITE LUNCH

Serves one.

⅛ pound sliced turkey breast from deli
2-ounce slice of hot pepper jack cheese
½ pound marinated mushrooms (from deli)

½ cup coffee served with ½ cup boiled low-fat
   milk
2 Pepperidge Farm Brussels cookies

EUROPEAN LUNCH

1 broiled chicken from supermarket
Small selection of cheeses, including Laughing
   Cow Reduced Calorie, Fontina, and whatever
   skim-milk cheese strikes my fancy—each person should have about 100 calories worth of
   cheese, probably three ¾-ounce pieces
Marinated vegetable salad (buy from deli, or
   make using recipe that follows)

Frozen fruit ice for dessert

MARINATED STRING BEAN SALAD

Serves two.

½ pound fresh string beans, Chinese long green
   beans, or haricots vert
¼ cup red wine vinegar
2 tablespoons olive oil
Garlic powder

   1. Cut beans into one-inch pieces, clean, and
steam until just cooked (al dente).
   2. Mix vinegar, oil, and garlic powder to make
dressing.

3. Marinate beans in dressing in refrigerator for at least one hour; overnight is better. Drain marinade to serve. Serve cold.

SUZY'S CHOPPED SALAD

Serves two.

½ head lettuce, limestone or Boston
½ head lettuce, red leaf
4 plum tomatoes (or 2 medium tomatoes)
3 ounces diet mozarella cheese
½ bunch cilantro
4 ounces garbanzo beans

1. Chop each ingredient separately, except for garbanzo beans. (I find them too hard to chop, so serve whole, unless you *want* to chop them.)
2. Mix chopped ingredients; add garbanzo beans.
3. Mix with dressing.

Dressing
Red wine vinegar
1 tablespoon olive oil
2 tablespoons lemon juice
1 tablespoon Dijon-style mustard
1 tablespoon plain, low-fat yogurt

1. Using Good Season or other marked cruet, fill red wine vinegar as directed to V line. Add water to W as directed, then add oil, lemon juice, mustard, and yogurt.
2. Shake well.
3. Mix yogurt in with straw if it is lumpy. Shake again.

Light dessert or fresh fruit (berries).

Dinner

In preparing my dinners for the week, I use a chart I have duplicated ad infinitum, which I keep stacked in the kitchen. Once a week I fill it out and attach it to the refrigerator door. This helps avoid the "What am I going to fix for dinner?" dilemma; allows me to do the shopping once or twice a week rather than daily; lets Mike know what's for dinner so he can make a contrasting lunch choice; and keeps us from eating too much meat, something I must always watch out for.

Once a week we eat lamb chops; once a week we go out; usually we go out one night of the weekend with our son. That means I only plan four dinners a week, which is fine by me. Like everyone else, I tend to make the same things over and over again, using the same ingredients on different types of foods. Below you'll find my basic month's worth of recipes, although I don't consign a dish to each day and may repeat some things as often as once a week. Others, I may do just for guests or when I get bored. None of them is hard, I promise.

You do not need to stick to these meals to lose weight, nor do you need any special cookbooks or charts. If each meal you serve totals 500 calories per person and your man does not drink more than two drinks a day, he will lose weight. Just make sure he eats a well-rounded 500 calories.

	SUNDAY	MONDAY	TUESDAY
DINNERS for the week of _____			
WEDNESDAY	THURSDAY	FRIDAY	SATURDAY

CHERRIED HEN

Serves two.

2 rock cornish hens, defrosted
1 cup chicken broth, canned
2 tablespoons lemon juice
Garlic, sage, poultry seasoning to taste
½ cup canned cherries, drained of syrup and rinsed in cold water
¼ cup grape juice

1. Place hens in baking pan. Pour ½ cup of the chicken broth over them.

2. Brush hens with lemon juice, then season to taste.

3. Bake in 325° oven, basting occasionally with remaining broth. Hens should always be standing in some liquid. Bake 45 minutes or until tender and golden brown. Remove skin after cooking.

4. Prepare sauce by heating cherries and grape juice until cherries are soft. You may have to add a teaspoon of water every now and then.

5. Place each hen on dinner plate, then spoon cherry sauce over it.

I serve with brown rice and a steamed vegetable; a light dessert.

HUNGARIAN CHICKEN

Serves four.

1 small onion, diced
2-pound frying chicken, cut up into pieces
1 6-ounce can of tomato or vegetable juice
⅓ cup old white wine (or cooking wine)

¼ pound mushrooms, sliced
Seasonings to taste (garlic powder, paprika, pepper, salt substitute)
2 tablespoons flour
½ cup plain, low-fat yogurt

1. Spray skillet with PAM; brown onion. Add chicken pieces and brown them,
2. Add juice, wine, mushrooms, and seasonings. Cover and simmer 30–35 minutes.
3. Remove chicken from skillet and broil until slightly crisp, about 10 minutes. Save liquid in skillet.
4. While chicken pieces are broiling, combine the flour and the yogurt in a small mixing bowl. Stir well to eliminate lumps. Then add to sauce in skillet, mixing well.
5. Remove chicken from broiler, place on dinner plates, spoon over sauce.

I serve this on a spoonful of egg noodles, or with one boiled potato per person and a vegetable, plus dessert.

BAR-B-Q CHICKEN

Serves 2–4.

1 chicken combo pack, or chicken parts per your taste (breasts preferred—one breast per person)
¼ cup store-bought barbecue sauce
1 8-ounce can vegetable juice or Snap-E-Tom
Dash of lite soy sauce or Tamari sauce
1 tablespoon red wine vinegar
1 tablespoon Dijon-style mustard
Garlic powder or fresh-ground garlic to taste

1. Remove skin from chicken parts.

2. Combine liquid ingredients and mustard in baking pan. Place chicken parts in liquid marinade, refrigerate overnight. (Cover with foil or wrap.)

3. First thing the next morning, turn the chicken parts over in the marinade.

4. Before cooking, sprinkle garlic powder or fresh ground garlic on the chicken pieces as you remove them from the marinade. Dispose of marinade.

5. Chicken tastes best when cooked on outdoor grill, but will broil almost as nicely.

I serve with corn on the cob and a salad and dessert.

RASPBERRY FISH

Garlic and other seasonings to taste
1 large fillet of fish per person (sole or sea bass, or try others)
1 large bundle of fresh spinach per person, chopped (1 box frozen chopped will do for each two people)
¼ cup lemon juice
Handful of raspberries (fresh) per person
1 lemon slice per person

1. Season fish to taste, and broil.

2. While fish is cooking, steam the spinach, but do not overcook. Should still be bright green.

3. When fish is done, place a bed of spinach on each dinner plate. Lay fish on top of the spinach, carefully so the fish does not crumble.

4. Quickly place lemon juice in small skillet and warm fresh raspberries. Do not allow them

to get mushy. Pour raspberry-lemon juice over fish and serve. Garnish with lemon slice.

That's a whole dinner as far as I'm concerned. Add salad if you want and/or dessert.

DILLY MEATBALLS

1 green onion per person, chopped
Fresh parsley, chopped
¼ pound ground veal per person (variation—use ground turkey or chicken*)
Fresh dill
Garlic and other seasonings to taste
3 tablespoons plain, low-fat yogurt per pound of meat

1. Chop green onion and parsley.
2. Combine ground veal, onion, parsley, dill, seasonings, and yogurt in mixing bowl.
3. Moisten hands with hot water. Do not shake them off so that as you work with the meat, some of the water mixes with the meat. Mix ingredients by hand and wooden spoon. When thoroughly mixed, wet hands again and form small meatball, about the size of a silver dollar. Count as you go so you come out with the same number of meatballs for each person.
4. Spray skillet with PAM. Brown meat balls.

Serve with rice pilaf, kasha, or bulgur wheat and a vegetable, plus dessert.

*When I prepare this dish as a chickenburger, I make larger patties and serve a sauce that is 3 tablespoons of plain, low-fat yogurt to each 1 tablespoon of Dijon-style mustard.

192

SHERRIED LIVER

Serves one. (I hate liver.)

½ small onion or 2–3 green onions, chopped
1 carton of chicken livers (between ¼–½ pound)
½ cup beef broth
¼ cup sherry

1. Brown onions in large saucepan or dutch oven.
2. Rinse livers and add to onions.
3. Cook in the beef broth on medium heat. Check occasionally to make sure liquid is not all cooked away. Add small amounts of water to keep moist.
4. When livers are just about done (about 20 minutes), add sherry and cook it down.

I serve this with two vegetables and dessert.

PASTA WITH STUFF

You can use any fresh vegetable combination you choose—I usually go with mushrooms and broccoli, but you can get creative. I also use either bow ties or curly pasta, but any kind will do.

½ cup mushrooms per person, sliced
1 head of broccoli
2 ounces of pasta per person
Garlic to taste (preferably fresh crushed garlic)
1 tablespoon oil

1. Slice mushrooms. Trim 4–6 flowers per person from the broccoli. Steam them slightly. They

193

should be bright green and al dente. Do not overcook.

2. Boil pasta in unsalted water.

3. While pasta is cooking, sauté steamed broccoli florets and sliced mushroom in skillet sprayed with PAM. Season with garlic. Brown veggies and garlic.

4. Pour cooked pasta into mixing bowl, toss in vegetables with oil. Serve while still hot.

CHICKEN ENCHILADA

I do this in my neighbor's microwave because it's so amazingly quick, but it works in an oven too.

1 corn tortilla per person
½ cup shredded, diet mozzarella cheese per person
1 cooked, skinless breast of chicken per person cut into bite-sized pieces, or shredded (leftovers are perfect)
2 tablespoons store-bought Salsa per person

1. Spray small skillet with PAM and quickly "fry" both sides of a tortilla.

2. Remove tortilla from skillet, place on microwave-proof cooking dish. Mix most of the cheese with all of the chicken and put on top of the tortilla, then roll it closed. Top with remaining cheese and the salsa.

3. Heat in microwave about 2 minutes until cheese is melted and bubbly. Or bake in 350° oven about 15 minutes, until cheese is melted and bubbly.

Serve with a grated lettuce salad and gazpacho, then serve sherbet for dessert.

194

STUFFED TROUT

1 small trout per person
½ cup cooked, cleaned, baby shrimp per person
¼ cup diced zucchini per person
2 tablespoons shredded, diet mozzarella cheese
1 tablespoon pine nuts (optional)
Seasonings to taste

1. Ask market to clean and prepare trout for stuffing. (I have head and tail removed at the store.)
2. Combine other ingredients in a mixing bowl; season to taste.
3. Place cleaned trout in foil-lined baking dish that has been sprayed with PAM. Stuff trout. Bake at 325° for 20–25 minutes or until fish is done.

If it looks too meager to satisfy your man, steam some more zucchini and add to the top of the cooked fish just before serving. Zucchini is low in calories, so fill him up with veggies. Sometimes I add a broiled tomato half to this—it also helps fill out the plate.

CHINESE CHICKEN SALAD

Serves two.

¼ cup peanut butter (crunchy preferred)
1 tablespoon peanut oil
1 teaspoon hot sesame oil
2 tablespoons lite soy sauce or Tamari
3 tablespoons water
1 diced scallion

1 tablespoon ground ginger
2 cups shredded, cooked chicken breast (leftovers are perfect)
1 bunch cilantro, chopped
1 head iceberg lettuce

1. Stir peanut butter into liquid ingredients (add water slowly). Add diced scallion and ginger; stir.

2. Add chicken and cilantro to dressing and stir, to coat.

3. Shred or chop lettuce and make into mound in center of dinner plate. Top with chicken mixture; toss lightly.

That's the whole dinner; serve fortune cookie for dessert or a creamy sherbet.

MAGIC PANCAKES

Serves three.

Crepe Batter
2 tablespoons butter
1 small onion, pureed in food processor
2 cups sliced mushrooms
¾ cup flour
¾ cup low-fat milk
2 eggs
1 teaspoon oil

Filling
1 cup sliced mushrooms
1 cup broccoli florets
½ cup chopped cilantro
Garlic to taste

Topping

1 heaping tablespoon plain, low-fat yogurt per crepe, mixed with chopped cilantro and fresh dill.

1. Make batter: Melt butter in a skillet (or margarine), add onion and mushrooms. Brown. Remove from heat.
2. In a mixing bowl, mix flour, milk, eggs, and oil until smooth. Add onion/mushroom mixture to mixing bowl; blend by hand.
3. Spray small skillet with PAM and spoon enough crepe batter to cover bottom. When mixture bubbles, turn with spatula. Make six crepes; warm in oven.
4. Make filling: While crepes are warming, stir-fry remaining mushrooms and broccoli florets in the same skillet, seasoning with cilantro and garlic.
5. Remove crepes from oven. Stuff with mushroom mixture; roll. Serve with dollop of plain lowfat yogurt mixed with chopped cilantro and fresh dill.

Just add dessert.

VEAL MEDALLIONS/AUNT LYNN

1 sliver butter per person
½ lemon per person, squeezed
2 shallots per person, diced
¼ cup cooking sherry or port
3 thin slices of veal scallopini per person (approximately .29 pound each)
Garlic powder and pepper to taste

1. Melt butter in skillet; add the lemon juice.
2. Sauté diced shallots in the juice. As the liquids cook down, add sherry gradually.
3. Sauté the veal, season with garlic and pepper to taste.

I serve with a steamed fresh vegetable and either brown rice or a new potato tossed with ½ teaspoon of inexpensive caviar. Boil the potato, slice or dice it. Mix the potato pieces with the caviar in a mixing bowl. If the caviar does not stick to the potato, add a drop of cooking oil. Toss and serve. You can also sprinkle a few parsley flakes. Add dessert.

CHICKEN CURRY

Serves 4–6.

1 cup plain, low-fat yogurt
½ 8-ounce can chicken stock
1 small onion, pureed in food processor
3 tablespoons curry powder
1 boned-and-skinned chicken breast per person
3–4 carrots, peeled and diced
1–2 turnips, peeled and diced

1. Mix yogurt, stock, and onion in a mixing bowl, and stir until blended.
2. Add curry powder and stir well. (Add or diminish amount of curry to personal taste.)
3. Place mixture in dutch oven or casserole; add chicken breasts and vegetables. Cover.
4. Bake in 350° oven for 45 minutes or until chicken is cooked. Check periodically to make sure there's enough liquid—add other ½ can of chicken broth or small amounts of water if needed.

Serve with brown rice; add dessert.

MOM'S LASAGNA (REVISED)

Serves six.

12 lasagna noodles
 1 zucchini, diced
 1 8-ounce can low-sodium, stewed tomatoes, drained and chopped
 1 8-ounce carton low-fat cottage cheese
 1-ounce package diet mozzarella cheese, shredded
 8 ounces tofu, diced
 1 medium onion, chopped finely
 1 28-ounce jar store-bought lite spaghetti sauce (or make your own)
Italian seasonings to taste

1. Cook the noodles and drain.
2. Spray baking pan with PAM. Line the bottom of the pan with four cooked noodles.
3. Sprinkle some of the zucchini, some of the tomatoes, and some of the cottage cheese across the noodles, forming a layer of ingredients.
4. Sprinkle some of the diet mozzarella cheese and the tofu.
5. Make a second layer, with noodles; then sprinkle more of the ingredients.
6. Make a third and final layer. Finish the ingredients. Then add the onion to the top. Top with the spaghetti sauce. Sprinkle on Italian seasonings.
7. Bake in 350° oven for 30–40 minutes.

That's the whole meal; serve with a small salad and a light dessert.

PASTA WITH TOMATO CREAM SAUCE

Serves two.

4 ounces linguini
1 8-ounce carton plain, low-fat yogurt
½ cup low-fat cottage cheese
2 tablespoons low-fat milk
1 tablespoon grated Parmesan cheese
1 4-ounce can vegetable juice or Snap-E-Tom
Garlic, seasonings to taste

1. Cook pasta until al dente.
2. While pasta is cooking, blend yogurt, cottage cheese, and milk in food processor or blender until more or less smooth.
3. Put mixture into mixing bowl, stir in Parmesan cheese, and add juice, Stir. Season to taste.
4. Drain cooked linguini, toss quickly in mixing bowl to coat with sauce. Serve immediately.

I serve with a small salad and dessert. You can add steamed vegetables on top if you need to serve more food—try a mixture of carrots and broccoli florets. Don't overcook the vegetables, please.

CHICKEN WITH CHEVRE

1 ounce Chevre (goat) cheese per person
1 sprig cilantro per breast, cut in tiny pieces
   with scissors
1 boned-and-skinned chicken breast per person
¼ cup cooking sherry (per 4 breasts)
2–3 shallots (per four breasts)

1. With a fork, mash together the cheese, chopped shallots and the cilantro.
2. With a mallet, flatten each chicken breast.

200

3. Poke several sets of holes in each breast with the tines of a dinner fork. Then coat each breast with a dab of sherry. Spread approximately one ounce of the cheese mixture on each breast.

4. Cover the breasts with wax paper, tap with the mallet once more. Refrigerate for 30 minutes.

5. Broil, cheese side up, for about 20 minutes, or until cooked.

I serve with brown rice or a boiled new potato (with caviar—see p. 198) and a steamed vegetable plus dessert.

VEAL CHOPS

About 5 each, per person, of three types of mushrooms if available in your market (I use shitake, oyster, and enoki.)
Garlic to taste
2 tablespoons plain low-fat yogurt
2 tablespoons Dijon-style mustard
¼ cup sherry
2–3 shallots, diced
1 large veal chop per person

1. Clean, and slice or chop the mushrooms. Spray skillet with PAM and sauté the mushrooms with fresh garlic until brown. Put aside.

2. Mix yogurt, mustard, and sherry until smooth.

3. In a skillet sprayed with PAM, sauté shallots, then add yogurt, sherry, and mustard mixture, which will just coat the bottom of the pan. Cook veal chops in mixture, turning twice to keep coated and to keep from burning. Add some sherry if liquid dries up. Cooking takes 5–8 minutes. Turn off heat.

4. Quickly toss mushroom mixture over the chops and sauce. Turn chops once and serve. Scoop up sauce and mushrooms and divide among the chops.

This is nice with rice pilaf, steamed veggies, and dessert. One veal chop is not much to eat, so you may want to serve with two steamed veggies—although there should be a nice-sized mound of mushrooms on top of the chop. Veal chops are outrageously expensive, so I use that as an excuse for not serving two per person.

TABOULI

Serves three or four.

2 cups boiling water
1 cup bulgur wheat
1 medium cucumber
2–3 medium tomatoes
1 cup broccoli florets
½ cup diced and peeled jicama
1 pound shrimp, cooked and cleaned (I buy from fish market already cooked)
1 bundle parsley
1 bundle cilantro
¼ cup lemon juice
1 tablespoon olive oil
2 tablespoons red wine vinegar
½ cup diced, diet mozzarella cheese
handful of pine nuts

1. Pour boiling water over bulgur in mixing bowl and let sit for one hour.
2. Chop vegetables, leaving broccoli florets in bite-sized pieces. Cut shrimps into three pieces

each. I use scissors for cutting parsley and cilantro, eliminating big stems, but using little stems.

3. When bulgur is "done," drain remaining water.

4. Add all vegetables, pour in liquids, and mix. Add pine nuts and cheese bits. Chill before serving.

Bulgur wheat has 600 calories per cup, so this meal can become calorie-heavy in no time at all. I bulk it up with lots of veggies and crunchies.

SUZY'S CHICKEN SALAD

1 cooked, boneless, skinless chicken breast per person

½ cup haricots verts (get in specialty market or use string beans or long beans) per person, steamed al dente and cut bite size

1 can artichoke bottoms (not in oil) per 4 servings, cubed

1 cup mushrooms, sliced

½ cup shitake mushrooms (if available—or another fancy mushroom), sliced

handful of pine nuts

1 8-ounce container plain, low-fat yogurt per 4 people

4–6 tablespoons Dijon-style mustard (to taste) per container of yogurt

1. Cut chicken into bite-sized pieces.

2. Mix chicken and all vegetable ingredients and pine nuts in large mixing bowl.

3. Mix yogurt and mustard in small bowl. Add to dry mixture.

Serve room temperature or chilled.

I make this in large quantities for dinner parties; it's also good in pita bread as sandwiches for lunch.

CHILI

Serves eight.

1 package chili spice mix (I use Wick Fowler's)
1 pound ground veal
1 pound ground turkey (or chicken)
1 medium onion, pureed in food processor
1 8-ounce can lite or low-sodium tomato sauce
1 package corn bread mix, prepared per directions

1. If your chili mix has onions and flour amongst them, eliminate those packets now. (Wick Fowler does.)

2. Brown the veal, turkey, and onion in large pan or dutch oven. Make sure meat is completely cooked before going on to next step. (Takes about 20 minutes.)

3. Add the spice packets, stir; then add tomato sauce. Bring to boil, stirring all the while.

4. Serve over 2-inch square of corn bread.

CHART HIS PROGRESS

Day One (date—_____):
Guestimate his current weight

Tell-All Day (date—_____):
You confess. He weighs in.

	100	125	150	175	200	225	250	275	300
Week One									
Week Two									
Week Three									
Week Four									
Week Five									
Week Six									
Week Seven									
Week Eight									
Week Nine									
Week Ten									
Week Eleven									
Week Twelve									

POUNDS

Place a dot or mark each week. Chart yourself in a different color ink.

205

MIKE'S AFTERWORD

Because she is an amazingly determined woman, my wife does what she says she's going to do. For that reason, I was only partly skeptical when she said she was going to make me a new man.

Well, Making Mike Marvelous turned out to be another of her successes. Not only did she do it, but the whole process was reasonably painless for me. I kept waiting for the moment when I'd blow up and cancel my subscription to my transformation, but it never came.

I actually found myself getting interested in nutrition for the first time. When I found I was still able to eat my homemade blend of cold cereal (see Mike's Mix. p. 182), I began to understand fully that it's not what you eat, but rather how much. When this revelation came, I felt like Einstein, relatively speaking.

I admit to a bit of backsliding, but going from 202 to 206 in two years isn't too bad, especially since I started at 238. In fact reading this book has stiffened my resolve. Stay tuned for Making Mike Marvelous II, and hang in there. You can do it. I did, with a little help from my friend. Thanks, Suze.

Michael Gershman
April 1984